Obstetrics and Gynecology

Obstetrics and Gynecology: PreTest® Self-Assessment and Review

Edited by
Alan H. DeCherney, M.D.

PreTest Service, Inc.
Wallingford

PreTest Service, Inc.: P.O. Box 330
71 South Turnpike
Wallingford, Connecticut 06492
(203) 265-5604

Editors: *Mary Ann C. Sheldon, Mark Schultz*
Editorial Assistant: *Donna D'Amico*
Typographer: *Elaine Reid*
Production Assistant: *Judith M. Raccio*
Artwork and Layout: *Robert Tutsky*
Cover Illustration: *"Confinement" by Maerten de Vos, courtesy of Yale Medical Library*
Cover Design: *Silverman Design*
Printer: *Hull Printing Company*

ISBN:0-914410-40-7

 Printed in the United States of America. Library of Congress Catalog Card Number: 77-78446.

Print Number: 9 8 7 6 5 4 3 2 1

Contents

List of Contributors

Richard L. Berkowitz, M.D.
Assistant Professor of Obstetrics & Gynecology and Public Health
Yale University School of Medicine
Medical Director
New Haven Chapter of Planned Parenthood League of Connecticut
New Haven, Connecticut

Donald R. Coustan, M.D.
Assistant Professor of Obstetrics & Gynecology
Yale University School of Medicine
New Haven, Connecticut

Alan H. DeCherney, M.D.
Assistant Professor of Obstetrics & Gynecology
Yale University School of Medicine
New Haven, Connecticut

Greggory R. DeVore, M.D.
Instructor of Obstetrics & Gynecology
Yale-New Haven Hospital
New Haven, Connecticut

Ronald S. Gibbs, M.D.
Assistant Professor of Obstetrics & Gynecology
University of Texas Medical School at San Antonio
San Antonio, Texas

Michael T. Mennuti, M.D.
Assistant Professor of Obstetrics & Gynecology
Fellow in Human Genetics
University of Pennsylvania School of Medicine
Philadelphia, Pennsylvania

William F. O'Brien, M.D.
Instructor of Obstetrics & Gynecology
Yale-New Haven Hospital
New Haven, Connecticut

Joel I. Polin, M.D.
Associate Professor of Obstetrics & Gynecology
Hospital of the University of Pennsylvania
Philadelphia, Pennsylvania

Peter E. Schwartz, M.D.
Assistant Professor of Obstetrics & Gynecology
Yale University School of Medicine
New Haven, Connecticut

Barney B. Silverman, M.D.
Assistant Clinical Professor of Obstetrics & Gynecology
Yale University School of Medicine
New Haven, Connecticut

John F. Steege, M.D.
Assistant Professor of Obstetrics & Gynecology
Duke University Medical Center
Durham, North Carolina

Lawrence J. Wartel, F.A.C.O.G., M.D.
Assistant Clinical Professor of Obstetrics & Gynecology
Yale University School of Medicine
New Haven, Connecticut

Introduction

Obstetrics and Gynecology: PreTest® Self-Assessment and Review has been designed to provide students, as well as physicians, with a comprehensive and convenient instrument for self-assessment and review within the field of obstetrics and gynecology. The 500 questions provided have the same format and are of the same degree of difficulty as the questions contained in Part II of the National Board of Medical Examiners examinations, the Federation Licensing Examination (FLEX), the Visa Qualifying Examination, and the ECFMG examination.

Each question in the book is accompanied by an answer, a paragraph explanation, and a specific page reference to either a current journal article, a textbook, or both. A four-page bibliography, listing all the sources used in the book, follows the last chapter.

Perhaps the most effective way to use this book is to allow yourself one minute to answer each question in a given chapter; as you proceed, indicate your answer beside each question. By following this suggestion, you will be approximating the time limits imposed by the board examinations previously mentioned.

When you finish answering the questions in a chapter, you should then spend as much time as you need verifying your answers and carefully reading the explanations. Although you should pay special attention to the explanations for the questions you answered incorrectly, you should read **every** explanation. The authors of this book have designed the explanations to reinforce and supplement the information tested by the questions. If, after reading the explanations for a given chapter, you feel you need still more information about the material covered, you should consult and study the references indicated.

This book should provide both an evaluative and educational experience; we also hope that you enjoy it. We would be very happy to receive your comments.

Obstetrics and Gynecology

Gynecology
General Considerations

William F. O'Brien

Lawrence J. Wartel

DIRECTIONS: Each question below contains five suggested answers. Choose the **one best** response to each question.

1. A 19-year-old woman comes to the emergency room and reports that she had passed out at work earlier in the day. She has mild vaginal bleeding and her abdomen is diffusely tender and distended. In addition, she complains of shoulder and abdominal pain. Temperature is 36.4°C (97.6°F); pulse rate, 120 per minute; and blood pressure, 96/50 mm Hg. To confirm the diagnosis suggested by the available clinical data, you now would perform which of the following diagnostic procedures?

(A) Dilatation and curettage
(B) Posterior colpotomy
(C) Pregnancy testing
(D) Culdocentesis
(E) Laparoscopy

2. Which of the following statements about ectopic tubal pregnancy is NOT true?

(A) Abdominal pain and bleeding are the most consistent findings
(B) The initial pain usually is intermittent and crampy
(C) The involved tube usually is grossly normal
(D) Amenorrhea is present in more than 90 percent of affected women
(E) Most abdominal pregnancies are "aborted" tubal pregnancies

3. A 43-year-old multiparous woman has a four-year history of irregular menses and frequent urination. Physical examination reveals an irregular uterus that is two or three times normal size. As the woman's physician, you now would

(A) perform a dilatation and curettage
(B) order a pregnancy test
(C) order ultrasonography
(D) order intravenous pyelography
(E) schedule a hysterectomy

4. Postpartum or postabortal pelvic inflammatory disease differs from gonorrheal pelvic inflammatory disease in all of the following respects EXCEPT

(A) the invasive quality of the organisms involved
(B) the vulnerability of the tissue to vascular spread
(C) the relative incidence of generalized sepsis
(D) the manifestations of the chronic phase of infection
(E) the potential for mortality

5. The condition that most often mimics true urinary stress incontinence is

(A) short urethra syndrome
(B) urethral diverticulum
(C) detrusor dyssynergia
(D) urgency incontinence
(E) overflow incontinence

6. The photomicrograph below represents a portion of uterine wall from a 43-year-old woman complaining of chronic pelvic pain and menorrhalgia that is unresponsive to hormonal therapy. The most likely diagnosis is

(A) endometriosis
(B) adenomyosis
(C) endometrial carcinoma
(D) ovarian carcinoma
(E) squamous cell carcinoma of the vulva

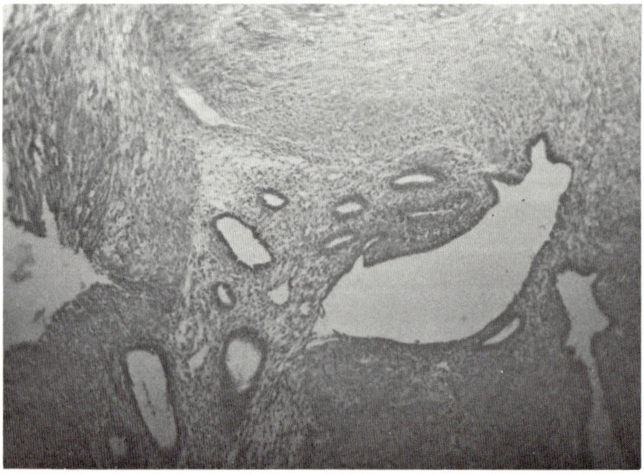

7. Which of the following statements about pelvic tuberculosis is true?

(A) The primary site of involvement is the endometrium
(B) Infertility is a late complication
(C) The diagnosis can be made by endometrial biopsy
(D) The PPD skin test is positive in about half of affected women
(E) Treatment often restores fertility

8. A 22-year-old woman, gravida 3, para 2 (one abortion), is brought to the hospital because she says she has been raped by a 35-year-old man whom she knows to have had a vasectomy two years ago. Both individuals have an A-positive blood type. Which of the following would be most useful to her in the prosecution of this case?

(A) Accurate description of the introitus
(B) Smear for sperm from the cervix
(C) Vaginal washings for acid phosphatase
(D) Specific typing of vaginal washings
(E) Examination of her pubic hair

9. The cause of ambiguous genitalia in about half of all affected infants is

(A) chromosomal nondisjunction
(B) gonadal dysgenesis
(C) adrenal hyperplasia
(D) mosaicism
(E) testicular feminization

10. A 42-year-old multiparous woman comes to your office complaining of irregular menses and frequent urination. Her pregnancy test is negative. Ultrasonography and physical examination suggest the presence of a fibroid uterus that is twice normal size. An examination performed six months earlier revealed a normal-size uterus. A hysterectomy would be recommended because

(A) a fibroid uterus can lead to abnormal bleeding
(B) a fibroid the size of a two-month pregnancy must be removed
(C) fibroids have a high malignant potential
(D) urinary frequency suggests severe pressure symptoms
(E) rapid appearance of fibroids warrants the procedure

11. Atypical adenomatous hyperplasia of the cervix has been associated with the use of oral contraceptives. Which of the following statements about this disorder is true?

(A) It develops within three months of initiation of oral contraception
(B) If left untreated, it usually progresses to a frankly malignant disease
(C) Mitotic figures are histologically common
(D) Lesions usually are friable and prone to bleeding
(E) Only the cells of endocervical glands are affected

12. Right ovarian vein syndrome is often associated with all of the following EXCEPT

(A) recurring right flank pain
(B) repeated episodes of right pyelonephritis
(C) cyclic hematuria
(D) premenstrual venous congestion
(E) appearance in women who have been pregnant at least once

13. A 22-year-old woman comes to your office for a labial sore that she first noticed two days ago. Physical examination reveals a small ulcer of the right labium majus. Until other information is available, which of the following disorders should be considered the primary diagnosis?

(A) Chancroid
(B) Primary syphilis
(C) Lymphogranuloma inguinale
(D) Herpes simplex infection
(E) Early carcinoma of the vulva

14. A 19-year-old woman comes to your office complaining of vague pelvic pain that is intermittent and aching and that is unrelieved by analgesics. Examination reveals several small lesions on the posterior fornix. Biopsy examination confirms the presence of endometriosis. Initial treatment should consist of

(A) radiation therapy
(B) induction of cyclic bleeding with estrogen and progesterone
(C) continuous therapy with a progestational agent
(D) excision of the lesions
(E) hysterectomy

15. All of the following statements about herpes genitalis are true EXCEPT

(A) affected women may present with urinary retention
(B) many affected women have accompanying trichomoniasis or *Hemophilus vaginalis* vaginitis
(C) primary infections can be asymptomatic
(D) recurrent lesions tend to be disseminated and conspicuous
(E) use of tricyclic dyes can shorten the clinical course

16. The ovarian cyst or tumor that is most common during infancy and childhood is

(A) dermoid cyst
(B) theca-lutein cyst
(C) giant follicle cyst
(D) granulosa cell tumor
(E) benign solid teratoma

17. Post-pill galactorrhea-amenorrhea syndrome commonly is associated with all of the following EXCEPT

(A) breast engorgement
(B) transient amenorrhea
(C) atrophy of the vaginal mucosa
(D) reduced levels of pituitary gonadotropins
(E) normal thyroid function

18. In the x-ray shown below, the small coalescent radiolucent areas within the uterus most likely represent

(A) cervical polyps
(B) interligamentous fibroids
(C) salpingitis isthmica nodosa
(D) carcinoma of the endometrium
(E) air bubbles

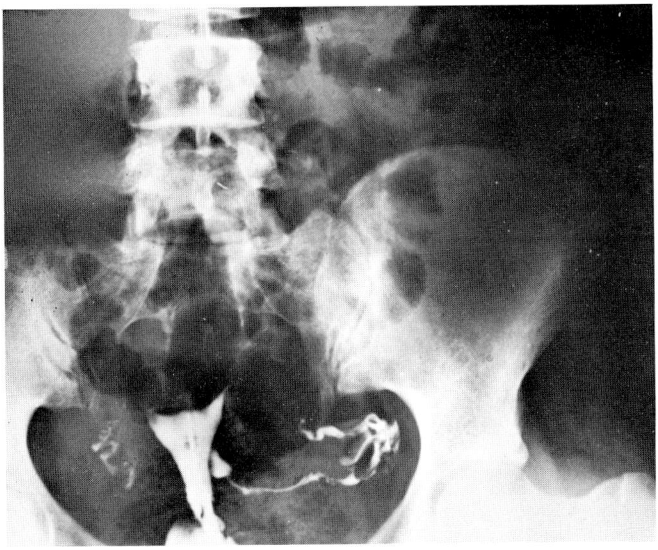

19. All of the following statements about endometriosis are true EXCEPT

(A) evidence of malignant changes is rare
(B) diagnosis usually can be established by history and physical examination
(C) although present in postmenopausal women, it is most common in women in their reproductive years
(D) affected women may present with infertility
(E) the most common site of involvement is the ovary

20. A 32-year-old woman, gravida 3, para 3, presents with abdominal pain. Her last menstrual period was six weeks ago, and a pregnancy test is positive. The specimen shown below is obtained at laparotomy. The most likely diagnosis is

(A) incomplete abortion
(B) missed abortion
(C) hydatidiform mole
(D) tubal ectopic pregnancy
(E) none of the above

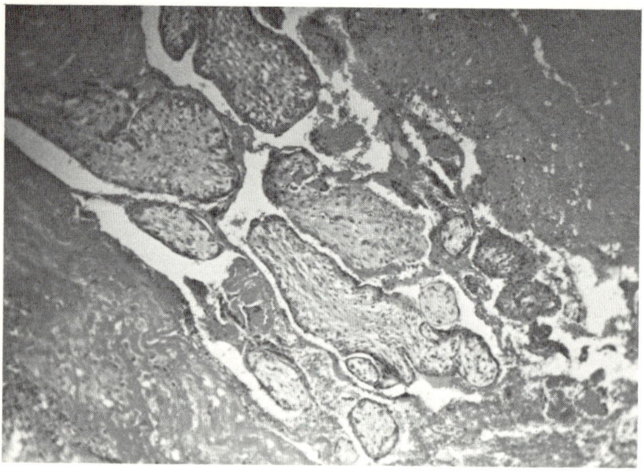

DIRECTIONS: Each question below contains four suggested answers of which **one** or **more** is correct. Choose the answer:

A	if	**1, 2, and 3**	are correct
B	if	**1 and 3**	are correct
C	if	**2 and 4**	are correct
D	if	**4**	is correct
E	if	**1, 2, 3, and 4**	are correct

21. Which of the following diagnostic procedures can be helpful in establishing the diagnosis of ectopic tubal pregnancy?

(1) Culdoscopy
(2) Laparoscopy
(3) Culdocentesis
(4) Colposcopy

22. At the present time, treatment of women who have endometriosis can consist of single-agent therapy with

(1) androgens
(2) progestational agents
(3) nonsteroidal gonadotropin inhibitors
(4) estrogens

23. Dermoid cysts of the ovary can be characterized by which of the following statements?

(1) They often are calcified and therefore are seen on abdominal x-ray
(2) They may be associated with severe "chemical" peritonitis if ruptured
(3) They are often pedunculated
(4) They are usually palpable posterior to the uterus

24. A 19-year-old woman consults you because of amenorrhea and galactorrhea of one year's duration. Her periods previously had been regular. She has had no other symptoms except for a mild headache. Computerized axial tomography of the head is ordered and the CAT scan is shown below. Diagnoses compatible with the findings on the CAT scan include

(1) empty sella syndrome
(2) amenorrhea of a nonpituitary etiology
(3) microadenoma of the pituitary gland
(4) suprasellar lesion of a pituitary adenoma

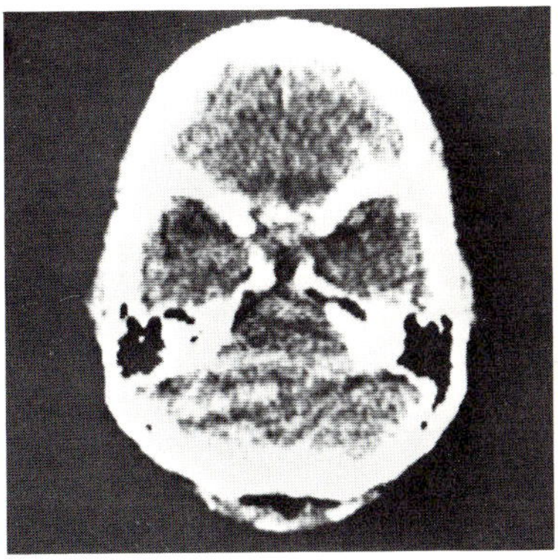

SUMMARY OF DIRECTIONS

A	B	C	D	E
1, 2, 3 only	1, 3 only	2, 4 only	4 only	All are correct

25. Gonococcal salpingitis is typically associated with which of the following?

(1) Unilateral abscess formation
(2) Lower-tract involvement of the urethra or Bartholin's gland
(3) Menstrual dysfunction, such as profuse bleeding, in the acute stage
(4) Pelvic tenderness in the absence of abdominal rigidity

26. The symptoms of endometriosis can include

(1) pain during defecation
(2) abnormal uterine bleeding
(3) dyspareunia
(4) progressive primary dysmenorrhea

27. Luteal-phase defect is associated with faulty ovulation. Which of the following studies performed in the second half of the menstrual cycle would be helpful in making a diagnosis?

(1) Serum progesterone levels
(2) Urine pregnanetriol levels
(3) Endometrial biopsy
(4) Serum luteinizing hormone levels

28. Albright's syndrome, a rare cause of isosexual female precocious puberty, is characterized by

(1) anovulatory uterine bleeding
(2) café au lait spots
(3) symmetric lesions of skin and bone
(4) gonadotropin secretion

29. Lymphogranuloma venereum, the incidence of which has been increasing in the United States, can be described by which of the following statements?

(1) It usually is accompanied by unilateral inguinal adenitis
(2) It can involve the anus, rectum, and sigmoid colon
(3) Affected women usually are unresponsive to penicillin
(4) Diagnosis by the Frei test is common

30. Hilus cell tumors of the ovary often are associated with

(1) increased excretion of 17-ketosteroids
(2) elevated levels of plasma testosterone
(3) elevated levels of 17-hydroxycorticoids
(4) hirsutism

31. Treatments commonly employed for women who have the vulvar lesion shown below include

(1) podophyllum
(2) 5-fluorouracil
(3) cryosurgery
(4) simple vulvectomy

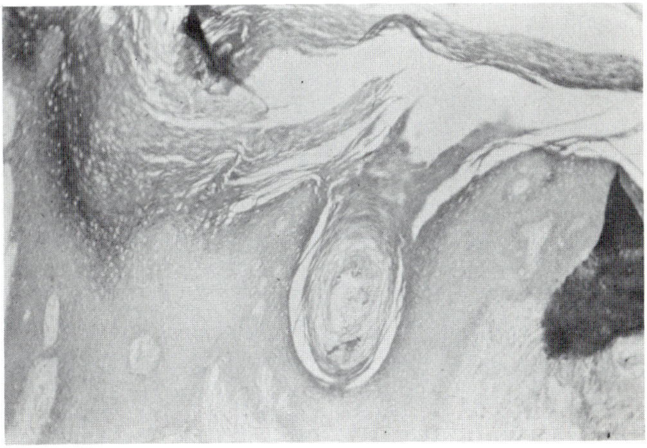

32. Recurring catamenial pneumothorax, which is a rare disorder of young women, can be described by which of the following statements?

(1) It usually is due to pleural endometriosis
(2) It can be inhibited by ovulation suppression
(3) It occurs with equal frequency on both sides of the chest
(4) It rarely is associated with underlying pulmonary pathology

33. Which of the following statements about clear cell adenocarcinoma of the cervix and vagina are true?

(1) It has been related to prenatal diethylstilbestrol exposure
(2) It shows a hobnail pattern on microscopic examination
(3) It usually appears as an exophytic lesion
(4) Affected women are best treated with radiotherapy

34. Histologic features that are diagnostic for endometriosis include

(1) endometrial glands
(2) evidence of hemorrhage
(3) endometrial stroma
(4) decidual reaction in the surrounding tissue

SUMMARY OF DIRECTIONS

A	B	C	D	E
1, 2, 3 only	1, 3 only	2, 4 only	4 only	All are correct

35. Which of the following statements about chancroid (soft chancre) are true?

(1) It is often accompanied by inguinal lymphadenopathy
(2) Diagnosis can be made by a complement fixation test
(3) Ducrey's bacillus (*Hemophilus ducreyi*) is the causative agent
(4) Affected individuals are best treated with a course of tetracycline

36. Gynecologists often are called upon to act as sexual counselors, marriage counselors, or both. Comparisons between unmarried women and married women reveal that

(1) married women have a higher incidence of phobias than unmarried women
(2) unmarried women have a higher incidence of depression than married women
(3) married women have a higher incidence of hypochondriasis than unmarried women
(4) married women are less apt to be dissatisfied with their jobs than unmarried women

37. The major pituitary hormones responsible for the luteal phases of the menstrual cycle are

(1) prolactin
(2) follicle-stimulating hormone
(3) luteinizing hormone
(4) growth hormone

38. The menopause invariably is accompanied by

(1) osteoporosis
(2) anxiety and depression
(3) cardiovascular degeneration
(4) decreased serum estrogen levels

39. The major estrogenic substances in postmenopausal women are

(1) estradiol
(2) estrone
(3) estriol
(4) androstenedione

40. The x-ray shown below reveals which of the following?

(1) Cornual obstruction
(2) Distended tubes
(3) Bilateral spill
(4) Bilateral hydrosalpinx

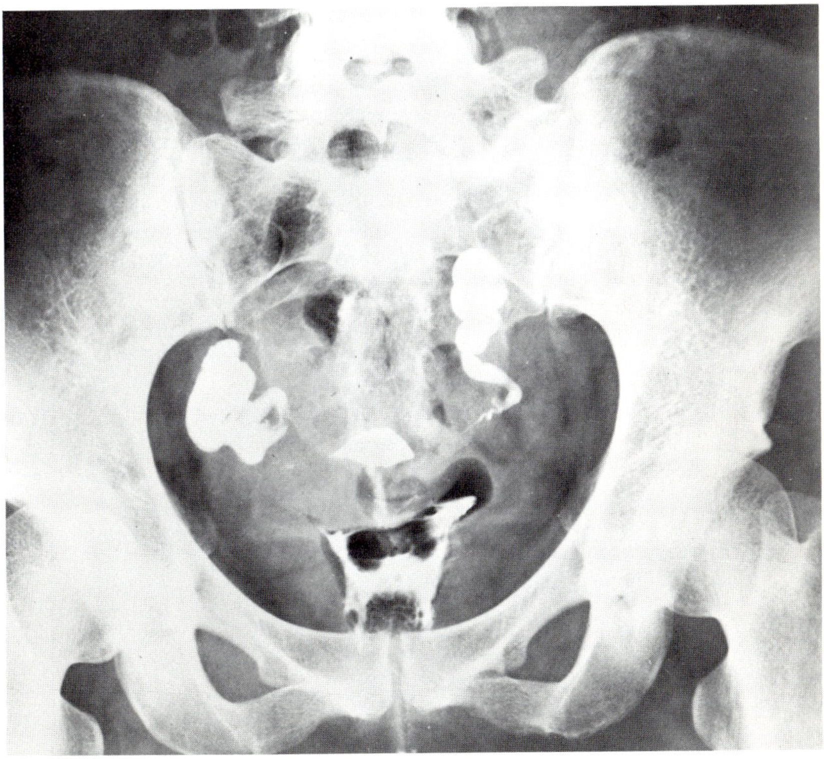

DIRECTIONS: The groups of questions below consist of lettered choices followed by several numbered items. For each numbered item select the **one** lettered choice with which it is **most** closely associated. Each lettered choice may be used once, more than once, or not at all.

Questions 41-44

For each clinical history given below, select the diagnosis with which it is most likely to be associated.

(A) Incomplete abortion
(B) Unruptured ectopic pregnancy
(C) Threatened abortion
(D) Persistent corpus luteum cyst
(E) Pelvic inflammatory disease

41. A 22-year-old woman, whose last menstrual period was five weeks ago, has had vaginal bleeding for nine days. She complains of pain in her lower abdomen, especially on the left side. Pelvic examination reveals moderate bleeding from a closed cervical os, a slightly enlarged uterus, and a tenderness in the left adnexa. Pregnancy test is negative

42. A 19-year-old woman, whose last menstrual period was seven weeks ago, reports that she has had vaginal bleeding for six days. In addition, she complains of severe lower abdominal cramps and lightheadedness. Pelvic examination reveals moderate bleeding from a patulous cervix. Pale tissue is noted in the posterior fornix. The uterus is slightly enlarged, and the patient notes mild tenderness in the region of the uterus and adnexa. Pregnancy test is negative

43. A 27-year-old woman, whose last menstrual period was six weeks ago, complains of having had vaginal bleeding and right-lower-quadrant pain for the last two weeks. Pelvic examination shows slight bleeding from a closed cervix. The uterus seems normal and there is a tender mass, 4 cm square, in the right adnexa. Pregnancy test is negative

44. A 25-year-old woman, whose last menstrual period was five weeks ago, says that vaginal spotting with bright red blood and lower abdominal cramps began five days ago. Pelvic examination reveals a closed cervix and slight bleeding. The uterus seems normal or slightly enlarged. Pregnancy test is read as doubtful for pregnancy

Questions 45-48

A 48-year-old woman enters the hospital for a total abdominal hysterectomy and bilateral salpingo-oophorectomy, which is performed on hospital day one. The woman's temperatures, recorded for her first eight days of hospitalization, are shown below. Realizing that postoperative pyrexia can stem from many causes, match the postoperative day with the therapeutic measure below that is most likely to be instituted during that day.

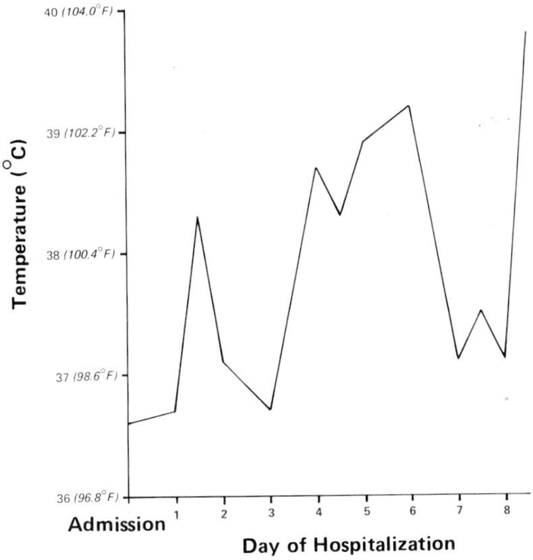

(A) Administration of heparin
(B) Administration of ampicillin
(C) Administration of chloramphenicol or clindamycin
(D) Intermittent positive-pressure breathing and deep-breathing exercises
(E) Vaginal or abdominal drainage

45. Day one (first night after surgery)

46. Day four

47. Day five

48. Day six

Questions 49-53

For each clinical description that follows, select the appropriate disorder.

(A) Neurogenic bladder
(B) Overflow incontinence
(C) Stress incontinence
(D) Vesicovaginal fistula
(E) Urgency incontinence

49. A 45-year-old woman states that she has had increasing difficulty holding urine after feeling the need to void. She occasionally loses urine when sitting down

50. A 43-year-old woman, who recently underwent an anterior vaginal repair, complains of constant perineal wetness and loss of urine while standing. She does not feel the urge to void

51. A 28-year-old diabetic woman reports that she loses large volumes of urine without warning. She says that she can overcome the problem by frequent, voluntary emptying of the bladder

52. A 26-year-old woman, who has four children, is worried because her daily jogging seems to be causing urinary dribbling

53. An 83-year-old woman, who lives in a nursing home, complains that dribbling of urine, which had occurred only when she was walking, now is markedly aggravated by a cold

Gynecology
General Considerations

Answers

1. **The answer is D.** *(Kistner, ed 2. pp 306-307.)* The clinical history presented in this question is a classic one for a ruptured tubal pregnancy accompanied by a hemoperitoneum. Because pregnancy tests are negative in almost half the cases, they are of little practical value in an emergency. Dilatation and curettage would not permit rapid enough diagnosis, and the results obtained by this procedure are variable. Culdocentesis is a rapid, nonsurgical method to confirm the presence of unclotted, intra-abdominal blood from a ruptured tubal pregnancy.

2. **The answer is D.** *(Green, ed 3. pp 290-293.)* The variability in clinical presentation of ectopic tubal pregnancy makes it one of the most difficult diagnostic problems in gynecology. Although tubal disease is an important etiologic factor, in most cases the tube is grossly and microscopically normal. Abdominal pain and vaginal bleeding are the most common symptoms. The pain, which is usually colicky and mild at first, later becomes intense and constant. In at least one-quarter of affected women, amenorrhea, which is considered to be characteristic of intrauterine gestation, does not develop. Tubal pregnancies that have "aborted" and become reimplanted are the most common cause of abdominal pregnancies.

3. **The answer is B.** *(Kistner, ed 2. p 231.)* If a woman in the child-bearing years has an enlarged uterus, a pregnancy test should be performed. Ultrasonography is a more expensive alternative; and an ultrasonogram may be difficult to interpret if fibroids and an intrauterine pregnancy both are present.

4. **The answer is D.** *(Green, ed 3. pp 256-269.)* The pathogenesis and presentation of postabortal or postpartum pelvic inflammatory disease, which is extremely life-threatening, differ in a number of respects from gonorrheal pelvic inflammatory disease. The relatively unprotected vessels of the gravid uterus are an easy portal for vascular entry of bacteria, which probably is a major reason for the increased incidence of generalized sepsis. The organisms responsible for these infections (gram-negative bacteria are the most common) are often more invasive and destructive than gonococci, which tend to spread superficially along the mucosa. In general, however, the manifestations of chronic infections and the management of affected women are similar.

5. **The answer is C.** *(Green, ed 3. pp 552-553.)* True urinary stress incontinence stems from the loss of normal muscular and endopelvic supports of a woman's pelvis. Correction of this condition lies in the reconstruction of these supports. In the evaluation of women suspected of having stress incontinence, other types of urinary dysfunction must be considered. Detrusor dyssynergia most often mimics true urinary stress incontinence; in many affected women, bladder emptying, triggered by an increase in intra-abdominal pressure, may resemble the leakage of urinary stress incontinence. Urethral diverticula, though they may be similar in appearance to cystourethroceles, are not associated with incontinence. Short urethra syndrome results in continuous leakage of urine, and urgency incontinence results in sudden, unrestrainable micturition.

6. **The answer is B.** *(Novak, ed 7. pp 261-271.)* The histologic and historical evidence presented in the question suggests adenomyosis. Adenomyosis is defined as endometrial tissue outside of the endometrial cavity and confined to the uterine wall. Tufts of endometrial tissue can be surrounded by areas of smooth muscle (myometrium), as in the accompanying photomicrograph. Endometriosis is defined as endometrial tissue outside of the uterus. Because the lesion shown is certainly benign, ovarian carcinoma and carcinoma of the vulva are ruled out. Women who have adenomyosis suffer from chronic pelvic pain and menorrhalgia, usually associated with an enlarged uterus. A diagnosis is rarely made clinically and usually depends on pathologic examination.

7. **The answer is C.** *(Green, ed 3. pp 270-272.)* The primary site of pelvic tuberculosis is the fallopian tubes. Although the endometrium is only secondarily affected, endometrial biopsy often is the easiest method of diagnosis. The tuberculin skin (PPD) test usually is positive. In view of primary tubal involvement, infertility is an early manifestation; and even with proper treatment, affected women have only a poor chance of regaining their childbearing capacity.

8. The answer is C. *(American College of Obstetricians and Gynecologists, ACOG Tech Bull 14[1972]: July.)* Although all of the procedures mentioned in the question can be helpful in establishing a case of rape in most situations, the expected lack of sperm and the matching blood types in the situation presented would limit their value in this case. Only the finding of 50 units/ml or more of acid phosphatase in this woman's vagina could be taken as evidence of ejaculation. Her introitus probably would not be injured because of her parity. Foreign pubic hair might only indicate close contact.

9. The answer is C. *(Green, ed 3. p 109.)* Although congenital adrenal hyperplasia affects both sexes, it more often is recognized in female infants. It accounts for approximately half of all cases of ambiguous sexual differentiation. Despite its genetic origin, congenital adrenal hyperplasia is not associated with karyotypic abnormalities. The most typical abnormality of external genitalia is clitoral enlargement, which is usually accompanied by some degree of hypospadias and labioscrotal fusion.

10. The answer is E. *(Kistner, ed 2. p 232.)* A rapid growth in fibroids is considered a valid indication for hysterectomy. Fibroids have a low malignant potential, rarely cause significant pressure when small, and may not cause bleeding problems even when left untreated.

11. The answer is D. *(Green, ed 3. p 244.)* Atypical adenomatous hyperplasia of the cervix associated with oral contraceptives is most significant because it often is confused with adenocarcinoma of the cervix. In view of the polypoid, friable nature of the lesions, affected women often present with contact bleeding. The lesions are benign, and histologic examination shows gland-cell and reserve-cell hyperplasia without any of the characteristics, such as abundance of mitotic figures, of malignancy. Atypical adenomatous hyperplasia of the cervix most commonly develops in women who have used oral contraceptives for several years.

12. The answer is C. *(Green, ed 3. p 171.)* Right ovarian vein syndrome is a type of acquired menstrual pain. It usually appears in women who have been pregnant at least once. The cause is believed to be related to incompetence of the valves of the right ovarian vein that can result during pregnancy. The clinical course features recurring ureteral obstruction and subsequent recurring right flank pain and pyelonephritis; these symptoms are due to premenstrual venous pelvic congestion and enlargement of the right ovarian vein.

13. The answer is B. *(Kistner, ed 2. p 33.)* The gross appearance of genital ulcers may give little information about the underlying disease process. Primary syphilis, chancroid, herpes simplex, lymphogranuloma inguinale, and early vulvar carcinoma all may be associated with ulcerative lesions; in addition, the "classic" hard ulcer of syphilis may, in fact, be soft, and the soft lesion of chancroid, hard. Experience has shown that, until ruled out, syphilis must be considered the working diagnosis.

14. The answer is C. *(Romney, pp 888-893.)* Initial treatment of young women who have small endometrial lesions that do not produce significantly severe symptoms should consist of observation and mild analgesics. Hormone therapy, such as with estrogen or progestins, usually is begun if initial treatment has been unrewarding and surgery is not recommended; the object of hormone therapy is to suppress, not stimulate, cyclic bleeding, which tends to aggravate endometriosis. Small endometriomas can be resected without compromising a woman's child-bearing capacity; radical surgery, on the other hand, is appropriate only for women who are not contemplating pregnancy and who fail to respond to other treatments.

15. The answer is D. *(Romney, pp 936-938.)* Symptoms of primary herpes genitalis may be quite severe and include blisters, ulcers, excruciating pain, and urinary retention. However, studies have shown that a significant number of women who show no signs of herpes genitalis may have antibodies to herpes simplex virus type 2, the causative agent of the disease; this finding indicates that these women have had previous, asymptomatic infections. Recurrent infections, which occur commonly, are localized and often hard to identify. Treatment of affected women with tricyclic dyes and photodynamic therapy has been able to shorten the clinical duration of the disease.

16. The answer is A. *(Green, ed 3. pp 126-127.)* Different types of ovarian cancer predominate at different stages of a woman's life. For example, adenocarcinomas, which occur primarily in postmenopausal women, are very rare in infants and children. Benign solid teratomas and especially dermoid cysts, on the other hand, make up about half of the ovarian neoplasms affecting young girls. Giant follicle cysts and theca-lutein cysts also occur rather frequently and presumably are due to maternal gonadotropin stimulation. Granulosa cell tumors, which develop before puberty in about 5 percent of cases, can be a cause of precocious puberty.

17. The answer is B. *(Green, ed 3. p 207.)* Post-pill galactorrhea-amenorrhea syndrome probably results from an induced dysfunction of the hypothalamic-pituitary axis. It is characterized by breast engorgement and vaginal, uterine, and ovarian atrophy. The amenorrhea of affected women frequently is permanent, and the galactorrhea can persist for several years. Although levels of pituitary gonadotropins are reduced, other endocrine systems are unaffected.

18. The answer is E. *(Kistner, ed 2. pp 121-122, 311-314.)* The radiolucent areas on the x-ray shown represent air bubbles. They appear to be coming from holes in the intrauterine cannula. Cervical polyps are cervical, not uterine, in origin and therefore would not appear in the uterine cavity. Interligamentous fibroids are seen in the broad ligament and cannot be seen on hysterosalpingogram. Salpingitis isthmica nodosa is a tubal disease, and in this x-ray the tubes are normal. Carcinoma of the endometrium is a space-taking lesion that usually is ragged and appears on the endometrial cavity.

19. The answer is B. *(Romney, pp 883-885.)* Endometriosis, which most commonly involves the ovaries, is a disease of women in their reproductive years, especially between the ages of 30 and 40 years. The disease is usually benign and reversible. The definitive diagnosis of endometriosis rarely can be established short of surgery or diagnostic laparoscopy. Diagnosis is aided by the presence of vulvar, vaginal, or cervical lesions, which can be biopsied; palpable cul-de-sac nodules; and a history of dysmenorrhea.

20. The answer is D. *(Novak, ed 7. p 490.)* The photomicrograph accompanying the question shows villi within a tubular structure; the villi are easily identified by the presence of cytotrophoblasts. The diagnosis is tubal ectopic pregnancy. Molar pregnancy, incomplete abortion, and missed abortion also can be associated with the presence of villi; but these disorders usually result in vaginal passage and are not associated with intra-abdominal presentation.

21. The answer is A (1, 2, 3). *(Wynn, pp 101-104.)* Colposcopy is used to examine cervical and vaginal epithelium and would not be helpful in diagnosing a suspected case of ectopic pregnancy. Both culdoscopy and laparoscopy involve the insertion of an endoscope into the peritoneal cavity, the former through the posterior vaginal fornix and the latter through the umbilicus. Either procedure can aid in establishing a diagnosis of ectopic pregnancy. Culdocentesis, the insertion of a needle through the posterior vaginal fornix, can detect a ruptured ectopic pregnancy.

22. The answer is A (1, 2, 3). *(Green, ed 3. pp 342-344.)* The major hormonal agents used at this time in the treatment of women who have endometriosis are progestins and androgens. Hormonal therapy has proved especially useful for women whose symptoms are mild. Because pregnancy can lessen the severity of endometriosis, estrogen therapy was tried as a possible treatment; the incidence of side effects and complications proved to be quite high, however, and estrogens now are used only for treatment of women with breakthrough-type bleeding. Gonadotropin inhibition has recently become possible without the use of steroid therapy.

23. The answer is A (1, 2, 3). *(Kistner, ed 2. pp 397-398.)* Dermoid cysts, which usually "float" anterior to the uterus, are characteristically pedunculated. The contents of a ruptured cyst are extremely irritating and may cause dramatic signs of peritonitis if diagnosis is delayed. The calcified areas characteristic of dermoids have the appearance of teeth and must be differentiated from phleboliths.

24. The answer is A (1, 2, 3). *(Speroff, pp 107-109.)* The computerized axial tomography (CAT) scan shown depicts a coronal section of the skull; the midline spherical area represents the sella turcica. In this study, the sella turcica is perfectly symmetric and normal in size. In the empty sella syndrome, the sella is basically normal in configuration; a portion of arachnoid membrane herniates down through the diaphragm and compresses the active pituitary gland. Because microadenomas of the pituitary gland, which can produce prolactin and thus cause amenorrhea and galactorrhea, are usually less than 5 mm in size, they would not appear in the CAT scan shown. A suprasellar lesion of the pituitary gland would be larger than 5 mm and therefore would appear on most CAT scans.

25. The answer is C (2, 4). *(Kistner, ed 2. pp 288-294.)* Because salpingitis secondary to gonorrhea is most often a bilateral process, abscess formation is usually bilateral. Although onset after menses accompanied by mild dysfunctional bleeding often occurs, hemorrhage is rare. Symptoms such as dysuria or frequent urination may indicate involvement of the lower genital tract. Although pelvic nerves may be stimulated by the peritoneal irritation that can accompany salpingitis, muscle spasm, such as that associated with appendicitis, is rarely seen.

26. The answer is A (1, 2, 3). *(Romney, pp 888-889.)* Pain, which may take the form of dyspareunia or painful defecation, is a usual complaint of women who have endometriosis. Abnormal patterns of urinary bleeding probably result from local alterations due to ovarian involvement rather than from central hormonal dysfunction. Endometriosis is associated with acquired dysmenorrhea.

27. The answer is B (1, 3). *(Behrman, ed 2. pp 308-314.)* A short luteal phase is defined as ovulation with poor production of progesterone in the second half of the cycle. Progesterone levels at that time of less than 7 ng/ml are diagnostic. Endometrial biopsy also is crucial to the diagnosis of this defect, because the endometrium will be out of phase with the time of cycle. For example, a biopsy taken on day 26 of the cycle will resemble endometrium of day 24 because of decreased progesterone stimulation. Pregnanetriol is a breakdown product of 17-hydroxyprogesterone, and levels are not helpful in diagnosing this condition. Determination of the level of pregnanediol, which is a metabolic product of progesterone excreted in the urine, is a helpful test. Serum luteinizing hormone levels have no correlation with the presence of a luteal phase defect.

28. The answer is C (2, 4). *(Green, ed 3. p 133.)* Approximately half of all individuals who have Albright's syndrome (polyostotic fibrous dysplasia) exhibit precocious puberty. The disorder is characterized by flat, brownish skin lesions (café au lait spots) and areas of fibrous dysplasia and cystic degeneration of the long bones. Only one side of the body usually is involved. The etiology of precocity in affected girls is believed to be pituitary or hypothalamic; gonadotropin levels are elevated, and ovulatory cycles are noted.

29. The answer is E (all). *(Green, ed 3. pp 277-278.)* Although the etiologic agent of lymphogranuloma venereum is a filterable virus, treatment with sulfonamides, chlortetracycline, or chloramphenicol is usually effective in the early stages of the infection. The initial prodrome (including fever and malaise) is followed by unilateral inguinal adenitis, which progresses to bubo formation. Lymphatic spread can lead to involvement of the anus, rectum, or sigmoid. The Frei skin test usually can diagnose lymphogranuloma venereum. Although it is primarily a disease of women who live in regions having a warm climate, lymphogranuloma venereum is on the increase in the United States, in part due to the return of infected soldiers from Vietnam and neighboring countries.

30. The answer is C (2, 4). *(Green, ed 3. p 190.)* Hilus cell (pure Leydig cell) tumors are small, unilateral tumors of the ovary. They cause hirsutism and virilization by production of testosterone; levels of 17-hydroxycorticoids and excretion of 17-ketosteroids are not usually increased. Hyperplasia and luteinization of the ovarian stroma often occurs and leads to endometrial hyperplasia (in contrast to endometrial atrophy that often accompanies arrhenoblastomas).

31. The answer is B (1, 3). *(Novak, ed 7. pp 27-28.)* The lesion shown in the question is condyloma acuminatum, also known as a venereal wart; it is a squamous lesion caused by the papilloma virus. Hyperkeratosis often is noted. The treatment is local excision, cryosurgery, or podophyllum, which is a locally acting, mild antimetabolite. 5-Fluorouracil is a very potent antimetabolite, and simple vulvectomy is too expensive a surgical procedure for removal of this benign, self-limiting lesion.

32. The answer is C (2, 4). *(Green, ed 3. p 156.)* Recurring catamenial pneumothorax is a disorder of regularly ovulating women and can be prevented by therapy aimed at the suppression of ovulation. It only occurs during menses and is apparently due to alveolar rupture caused by an as yet unidentified sequela of normal ovulation. Examination of an affected lung shows little, if any, underlying pathology. In contrast to cyclic hemoptysis, recurring catamenial pneumothorax is not associated with endometriosis. The phenomenon is limited to the right thorax.

33. The answer is A (1, 2, 3). *(Green, ed 3. pp 128-131.)* In the late 1960's, a surprisingly large number of cases of a rare type of clear cell adenocarcinoma of the cervix and vagina were discovered in Boston. Careful epidemiologic investigation revealed that nearly all the mothers of affected girls had taken diethylstilbestrol or a similar drug during pregnancy. These tumors are exophytic lesions that are friable and red. Microscopic examination characteristically reveals the presence of cystic spaces lined with so-called hobnail cells. Because affected patients usually are in their adolescence and because the tumors are relatively radioresistant, surgery has been the main component of management.

34. The answer is A (1, 2, 3). *(Green, ed 3. p 334.)* In view of the importance of accuracy in diagnosing endometriosis, strict, definitive criteria must be used. The triad of histologic findings that is diagnostic for endometriosis consists of the presence of endometrial glands and endometrial stroma and evidence of recent or old hemorrhage. In women who are pregnant or who are receiving certain forms of hormonal therapy, a significant decidual reaction may be seen; this feature, however, is by no means diagnostic for endometriosis.

35. The answer is B (1, 3). *(Green, ed 3. p 277.)* Chancroid (soft chancre) is a very contagious venereal disease that is caused by *Hemophilus ducreyi*. Painful, tender lesions of the external genitalia usually appear three to ten days after a sexual encounter with an infected individual. Development of these lesions frequently is followed by enlargement of inguinal lymph nodes. Diagnosis is usually made by a culture of the ulcerated lesion; and treatment of affected individuals is with a two-week course of streptomycin or sulfonamides.

36. The answer is B (1, 3). *(Romney, pp 529-530.)* At least 40 percent of marriages end in divorce, and in most cases it is the wife, not the husband, who considers the marriage an unhappy one. Psychological and physical anxieties are both more common among married women than among married men. However, in a comparison of married and unmarried women, unmarried women were found to be far less subject to anxiety, depression, hypochondriasis, and job dissatisfaction. Unmarried women also were found to be healthier than unmarried men, as well as to have higher educational levels and higher average incomes.

37. The answer is B (1, 3). *(Green, ed 3. p 148.)* In the early part of the menstrual cycle, follicle-stimulating hormone seems to be the hormone responsible in large part for maturation of ovarian follicles. At midcycle there is a surge of luteinizing hormone, and high levels are sustained throughout the luteal phase. Secretion of prolactin, which probably aids in the luteinization of the follicle, also occurs at this time.

38. The answer is D (4). *(Wynn, p 166.)* The *sine qua non* of the menopause is ovarian failure; a marked decrease in estrogen production subsequently results, and a secondary increase in the production of follicle-stimulating hormone (FSH) by the pituitary is noted. Symptoms of emotional upset may be due more to a change in life situation than in hormonal balance. Cardiovascular and bony degeneration occurs in some, but by no means all, women. Estrogen replacement therapy is usually effective in relieving symptoms associated with menopause; its use is least effective in treating women who develop osteoporosis.

39. The answer is C (2, 4). *(Green, ed 3. p 567.)* During their reproductive years, the major estrogenic substance produced by women is estradiol. Pregnancy brings about an enormous rise in the level of estriol. With the cessation of ovulation, estradiol production falls, and production of estrone and androstenedione increases. Androstenedione is converted peripherally to estrone.

40. The answer is C (2, 4). *(Kistner, ed 2. pp 290-294.)* The x-ray presented reveals bilateral hydrosalpinx and distended tubes; no spill is noted at the fimbriated extremity. These findings are suggestive of chronic pelvic inflammatory disease. Both cornual areas appear normal, and there is no spill into the peritoneal cavity.

41-44. The answers are: 41-B, 42-A, 43-D, 44-C. *(Kistner, ed 2. pp 304-306, 347. Pritchard, ed 15. pp 489-490.)* Vaginal bleeding and lower abdominal pain following a delayed onset of menses can suggest any of the disorders presented. Standard pregnancy tests are rarely positive if onset of menses has been delayed for less than 15 days. Bleeding and cramping accompanied by no other significant symptoms suggest a threatened abortion; the presence of tissue and a dilated cervix, on the other hand, points to a diagnosis of incomplete abortion. Because symptoms of an unruptured ectopic pregnancy and a persistent corpus luteum cyst are so similar, the slight enlargement of the uterus that is sometimes associated with the former may be the only way to distinguish the two disorders. Definitive diagnosis of any of these disorders might require laparoscopy.

45-48. The answers are: 45-D, 46-B, 47-C, 48-E. *(Romney, pp 448-455.)* The hospital course of the patient described reflects many of the diagnostic situations that can face a clinician. A rapid rise in temperature in the early postoperative period often can be traced to atelectasis; pulmonary problems can be treated by using intermittent positive-pressure breathing and by getting the patient to cough and perform deep-breathing exercises. Early pelvic cellulitis, which is responsible for the rise on day four of the patient's temperature, should be treated initially with standard antibiotic therapy, including the use of such medications as ampicillin. Failure to respond in 24 to 48 hours should suggest the presence of an anaerobic infection; appropriate therapy with, for example, chloramphenicol or clindamycin, should then be instituted. Because *Bacteroides* infections are associated with a high incidence of pelvic abscess, failure of a patient to respond to appropriate antibiotic treatment should prompt a search for this condition. The patient's fever on day eight might indicate recollection of a pelvic abscess or pelvic thrombophlebitis, which also is often associated with anaerobic infections.

49-53. The answers are: 49-E, 50-D, 51-A, 52-C, 53-B. *(Romney, pp 268-271.)* Urgency incontinence resulting from hyperactivity of the detrusor muscle is associated with the loss of large amounts of urine just after a woman has had an urge to void. Sudden motions can trigger the urge.

Small fistulas can result from improperly performed surgery that has created an unnoticed entry into the bladder. Affected patients, when recumbent, will pool urine in the vagina.

Diabetes as well as neurologic disorders can be associated with neurogenic bladder. Reflex emptying, which usually is spasmodic and not accompanied by a sensation of a full bladder, is characteristic of the disorder.

Characteristically, stress incontinence is the loss of urine caused by sudden increases in intra-abdominal pressure. The condition is uncommon in women who never have been pregnant.

Conditions that cause pressure on or constriction of the bladder neck can lead to an overdistended bladder. Overflow incontinence also occurs not infrequently among elderly patients.

Gynecology Surgical Considerations

Greggory R. DeVore

DIRECTIONS: Each question below contains five suggested answers. Choose the **one best** response to each question.

54. The best landmark for determining where to separate the rectus muscles in a midline incision is the

(A) urachus
(B) umbilicus
(C) linea nigra
(D) pyramidalis muscles
(E) midline of the symphysis pubis

55. Which is the most common sign of impending evisceration from a wound incision?

(A) Serous drainage
(B) Sanguineous drainage
(C) Serosanguineous drainage
(D) Abdominal pain with no drainage
(E) Abdominal contents in the wound

56. A woman has been anuric for the first 48 hours after undergoing abdominal hysterectomy. Bilateral ligation of the ureters is suspected. Which of the following therapeutic measures should be ordered?

(A) Observation only
(B) Ureteral catheterization
(C) Rapid dialysis
(D) Transabdominal deligation
(E) Bilateral nephrostomy

57. The most important indication for surgical repair of a double uterus is

(A) habitual abortion
(B) dysmenorrhea
(C) menometrorrhagia
(D) dyspareunia
(E) premature delivery

58. All of the following statements concerning ectopic pregnancy are true EXCEPT

(A) it occurs more commonly among black women than white
(B) the fallopian tube is the most common site of implantation
(C) if a woman has had a tubal pregnancy or undergone tubal plastic surgery, the chance of having a future ectopic pregnancy is 10 to 20 times greater than in the general population
(D) one of the most important etiologic factors is pelvic inflammatory disease
(E) its incidence in women who have pelvic inflammatory disease is decreased by the use of conventional antibiotic therapy

59. Which of the following statements about the endometrial Arias-Stella reaction in pregnant women is NOT true?

(A) It was first described in association with tubal pregnancy
(B) It is a reaction of glandular epithelial cells
(C) It is a sign of impending fetal death
(D) Affected cells have abundant, eosinophilic-staining cytoplasm
(E) The nuclei of affected cells are hyperchromatic and increased in size

60. All of the following statements about abdominal pregnancy are true EXCEPT

(A) secondary implantations are more common than primary
(B) symptoms include abdominal discomfort and fetal movement in the abdomen
(C) it can be diagnosed by failure of oxytocin induction of labor
(D) ultrasound is a safe and effective means of diagnosis
(E) the placenta should be removed at the time of delivery to prevent eventual uncontrolled hemorrhage

61. The most common site of endometriosis is the

(A) uterine surface
(B) anterior cul-de-sac
(C) posterior cul-de-sac
(D) ovary—unilateral involvement
(E) ovary—bilateral involvement

62. Which of the following conditions is NOT an indication for abdominal surgery during the acute phase of salpingitis?

(A) A tubo-ovarian abscess that cannot be reached vaginally
(B) A fluctuant cul-de-sac abscess that is unresponsive to conservative (antibiotic) treatment
(C) Obstruction caused by an adherent loop of bowel
(D) Severe bilateral pain in the lower abdomen
(E) Severe right-lower-quadrant pain and tenderness

63. Differentiating between pelvic inflammatory disease and acute appendicitis can be difficult, because the two disorders can share all of the following symptoms EXCEPT

(A) nausea and vomiting
(B) intestinal obstruction
(C) generalized muscle spasms
(D) psoas-muscle tenderness
(E) abdominal pain in the suprapubic region

64. All of the following steps are appropriate in the management of a woman who has a ruptured tubo-ovarian abscess EXCEPT

(A) preoperative antibiotic coverage consisting of penicillin and an aminoglycoside
(B) preoperative blood transfusions
(C) rapidly performed surgery (subtotal hysterectomy)
(D) bilateral salpingo-oophorectomy
(E) constant postoperative intestinal suction

65. On the third postoperative day following pelvic surgery, a woman develops right costovertebral tenderness and a temperature of 38.9°C (102°F). A Gram stain of unspun urine obtained from a catheter specimen reveals gram-negative rods. Urine culture grows *Proteus mirabilis* sensitive to gentamicin. Despite treatment with 1.5 mg/kg of gentamicin, the woman continues to have pyelitic symptoms and a fever. Her physician now should

(A) discontinue the gentamicin
(B) increase the dose of gentamicin to 1.75 mg/kg
(C) add another antimicrobial agent, such as clindamycin or carbenicillin, that is effective against *Bacteroides fragilis*
(D) treat the patient with heparin
(E) catheterize the right ureter

DIRECTIONS: Each question below contains four suggested answers of which **one** or **more** is correct. Choose the answer:

A	if	**1, 2, and 3**	are correct
B	if	**1 and 3**	are correct
C	if	**2 and 4**	are correct
D	if	**4**	is correct
E	if	**1, 2, 3, and 4**	are correct

66. The advantages of transverse abdominal incisions include

(1) a decreased incidence of incisional hernias
(2) the requirement of only light general anesthesia
(3) a scar that can be cosmetically hidden
(4) easy access to the upper abdomen for bowel surgery

67. Indications for a gridiron (muscle-splitting) incision include which of the following procedures?

(1) Extraperitoneal drainage of a broad-ligament abscess
(2) Drainage of a tubo-ovarian abscess
(3) Drainage of the pelvis during a pelvic laparotomy
(4) Excision of a large ovarian cyst

68. Which of the following statements about myomata uteri are true?

(1) They arise mainly from fibrous tissue
(2) Pedunculation can be seen with submucous or subserous tumors
(3) They rarely cause bleeding
(4) Their excision is the most common indication for hysterectomy

69. During gynecologic surgery, operative injuries to the ureter occur

(1) more frequently in association with vaginal rather than abdominal hysterectomy
(2) only rarely if periureteral tissue is dissected carefully
(3) most commonly when the ureter lies between the anterior vaginal wall and the base of the bladder
(4) often as a result of hasty reclamping of vessel clamps or ligatures

70. If ureteral injury is recognized at the time of surgery, which of the following procedures could be recommended?

(1) A longitudinal slit should be made in the ureter below the injury and a polyethylene tube threaded into the bladder
(2) If the ureter is not severed, the site of injury should be drained intraperitoneally
(3) If the ureter is severed, uretero-ureteral anastomosis should be attempted, regardless of the location of the injury
(4) If possible, the severed ureter should be implanted into the bladder

71. Which of the following statements about interstitial tubal pregnancy are true?

(1) Its incidence increases in women who have had a salpingectomy
(2) It tends to rupture at an earlier stage than other tubal pregnancies
(3) A significant percentage can be diagnosed before rupture
(4) Rupture causes less blood loss than rupture of pregnancies in the ampullary portion of the tube

72. Indications for presacral neurectomy include

(1) primary or secondary dysmenorrhea that does not respond to medical management
(2) pelvic pain secondary to inoperable pelvic carcinoma
(3) conservative surgery for endometriosis
(4) dyspareunia

73. Which of the following statements about appendicitis during pregnancy are true?

(1) Premature labor occurs commonly
(2) Mortality rate is much higher in pregnant than nonpregnant women
(3) Symptoms may be mistaken for those classically associated with pregnancy itself
(4) It is frequently mistaken for pyelitis of the right kidney

DIRECTIONS: The group of questions below consists of lettered choices followed by several numbered items. For each numbered item select the **one** lettered choice with which it is **most** closely associated. Each lettered choice may be used once, more than once, or not at all.

Questions 74-77

For each description that follows, select the operative procedure with which it is most likely to be associated.

(A) Salpingoplasty
(B) Salpingostomy
(C) Salpingolysis
(D) Fimbriolysis
(E) Uterotubal implantation

74. Placing the uterine tube in a new opening created in the fundal portion of the uterus

75. Section of adhesions causing conglutination of the fimbria

76. Cutting adhesions around the uterine tube

77. Opening up a previously formed hydrosalpinx

Gynecology
Surgical Considerations

Answers

54. The answer is D. *(Te Linde, ed 4. pp 125-127.)* For separation of the rectus muscles in a midline incision, the pyramidalis muscles are the best landmark, because their medial borders insert into the linea alba in the midline. Although the other landmarks listed in the question are also in the midline, they are not reliable markers, because they either can vary in location or are not yet visible during the initial stages of surgery. Low midline incisions are the most common abdominal incisions for surgery on female reproductive structures.

55. The answer is C. *(Te Linde, ed 4. p 141.)* Serosanguineous drainage occurs very frequently before evisceration from an incision. Drainage can be accompanied by pain or by the feeling that something is "giving away." Serous or sanguineous drainage often is noted postoperatively and usually suggests involvement of the superficial wound.

56. The answer is B. *(Te Linde, ed 4. p 273.)* Bilateral ureteral obstruction, if unrecognized or unrelieved, can cause death in seven to ten days. Once the presence of bilateral ureteral obstruction is suspected, bilateral ureteral catheters should be passed in order to demonstrate and, if possible, overcome the obstructions. If obstruction persists, bilateral nephrostomy should be performed; if, six to eight weeks later, the obstructions still cannot be overcome, ureteral surgery should be undertaken.

57. The answer is A. *(Te Linde, ed 4. pp 284-285.)* Habitual abortion is the most important indication for surgical treatment of women who have a double uterus. The abortion rate in women who have a double uterus is two to three times greater than that of the general population. Therefore, women who present with habitual abortion should be evaluated by hysterosalpingography to detect a possible double uterus. Dysmenorrhea, premature delivery, dyspareunia, and menometrorrhagia are other, less important indications for surgical intervention.

58. The answer is E. *(Te Linde, ed 4. pp 323-324, 339.)* Ectopic pregnancy, which occurs most commonly in the fallopian tubes but also in the ovary, peritoneal cavity, and broad ligament, appears to be more common among black women than white women. The incidence of ectopic pregnancy seems to be increasing (although the mortality rate is decreasing); the incidence is especially high – 10 to 20 times that of the general population – in women who have had a previous tubal pregnancy or undergone tubal plastic surgery. Histologic evidence of pelvic inflammatory disease is found in a significant number of women who have had tubal pregnancies. However, this increase in the incidence of ectopic pregnancy in women who have pelvic inflammatory disease may be due to the antibiotics used to treat the disease, rather than the disease itself.

59. The answer is C. *(Te Linde, ed 4. pp 327-329.)* Although the Arias-Stella reaction was first described in association with tubal pregnancy, it can occur in association with any condition in which active chorial tissue is present; these conditions include abortions, syncytial endometritis, hydatidiform mole, and choriocarcinoma. The Arias-Stella reaction affects glandular epithelial cells of the endometrium. These cells have abundant, vacuolated, eosinophilic cytoplasm and enlarged, hyperchromatic nuclei. This endometrial-gland reaction occurs after fetal death.

60. The answer is E. *(Te Linde, ed 4. pp 336-340.)* Most authorities believe that the placenta should remain within the abdominal cavity following delivery of an abdominal pregnancy, because removal can lead to blood loss that can be quite difficult to control. If removal of the placenta is desired, it is best to wait until the placental vessels have fibrosed. Some investigators have treated affected women with methotrexate to speed up trophoblastic degeneration. A history of abdominal fetal movements and discomfort suggests abdominal pregnancy, which can be diagnosed by radiography, ultrasonography, failure of oxytocin to induce labor, or other means able to demonstrate the presence of a fetus in the abdomen. Most abdominal pregnancies stem from reimplantation of a ruptured or an aborted early tubal pregnancy.

61. The answer is D. *(Te Linde, ed 4. p 198.)* The most common site of endometriosis is the ovary; unilateral involvement is more than twice as common as bilateral involvement. Superficial serosal lesions also are common, especially on the uterine and tubal surfaces and in scattered locations on the pelvic serosa.

62. The answer is D. *(Te Linde, ed 4. pp 234-237.)* Unless absolutely necessary, abdominal surgery for women who have acute salpingitis should be postponed until after the infection has resolved. Operations performed during the acute phase of salpingitis are associated with increased rates of mortality and morbidity. Indications for surgery in affected women include drainage of persistent tubo-ovarian or fluctuant cul-de-sac abscesses, obstruction of the bowel caused by the adhesion of a loop of the small intestine, and a strong suspicion of acute appendicitis.

63. The answer is D. *(Te Linde, ed 4. pp 234-235.)* Differentiating between acute appendicitis and pelvic inflammatory disease can be a vexing diagnostic problem, because the symptomatology of the two disorders is very similar. Suprapubic abdominal pain, nausea and vomiting, intestinal obstruction, and generalized muscle spasms all can occur in both diseases. Tenderness of the psoas muscle, however, can be a helpful diagnostic sign, because the psoas muscle does not extend into the pelvis; therefore, right-lower-quadrant pain caused by the stretching of this muscle usually indicates appendicitis.

64. The answer is A. *(Te Linde, ed 4. p 243.)* An important aspect that is often overlooked in the management of a woman who has a tubo-ovarian abscess is preoperative antibiotic coverage for *Bacteroides fragilis*. Because penicillin combined with an aminoglycoside can cover all potential pathogens except *B. fragilis*, clindamycin, carbenicillin, or chloramphenicol should be added to the antibiotic regimen. Because patients are put in Trendelenberg position, rapid surgery is required; thus, a subtotal hysterectomy frequently is performed. For most patients, bilateral salpingo-oophorectomy also is indicated, and postoperative intestinal suction is recommended.

65. The answer is E. *(Te Linde, ed 4. pp 273-274.)* In a woman who has postoperative pyelitis, failure of costovertebral tenderness to disappear following appropriate antibiotic coverage suggests ureteral obstruction, and the appropriate ureter should be catheterized to demonstrate or, if possible, clear the obstruction. The presence of pelvic thrombophlebitis also should be considered but not before ureteral catheterization has ruled out obstruction. Because *Bacteroides fragilis* does not cause urinary-tract infections, use of antimicrobials effective against this organism is unnecessary.

66. The answer is B (1, 3). *(Te Linde, ed 4. p 128.)* Benefits of a low transverse abdominal incision are a decreased incidence of incisional hernias and cosmetic placement of the scar near the edge of the pubic hairline. The use of light anesthesia is contraindicated due to its poor muscle relaxation. Bowel surgery is best approached with a vertical incision, especially if a colostomy is anticipated.

67. The answer is A (1, 2, 3). *(Te Linde, ed 4. pp 131-132.)* Gridiron (muscle-splitting) abdominal incisions are effective for extraperitoneal drainage of an infection, such as a tubo-ovarian or broad-ligament abscess. If drainage of the abdominal cavity is necessary during a laparotomy, it is best to drain through a gridiron incision and not through the initial incision. An ovarian cyst should be approached through either a midline or low-transverse incision.

68. The answer is C (2, 4). *(Te Linde, ed 4. pp 143-151.)* Myomata uteri (uterine fibroids) arise from fibromuscular tissue, with more smooth muscle than fibrous tissue present. All myomata uteri arise in the myometrium; and although they initially occur interstitially, they can grow internally (submucous lesions) or externally (subserous) and become pedunculated. Myomata uteri, which frequently cause bleeding, are the most common uterine tumors; their excision, not surprisingly, is the most common indication for hysterectomy.

69. The answer is D (4). *(Te Linde, ed 4. pp 270-271.)* Operative injuries to the ureter are associated more commonly with abdominal hysterectomy rather than vaginal hysterectomy. The most common site of injury occurs near the region of the uterine vessels. Because the blood supply to the ureter arises from the periureteral tissue, dissection should be avoided; even careful dissection results in a significant percentage of ureteral injuries, and the incidence of fistula formation is increased if the blood supply is compromised. Slippage of vessels from clamps or ligatures can lead to ureteral injury if the vessels are reclamped hastily in an effort to stop the resultant bleeding.

70. The answer is D (4). *(Te Linde, ed 4. pp 272-273.)* Following injury to the ureter during surgery, a drain should be placed extraperitoneally. If a polyethylene catheter is inserted, it should be placed above the site of injury so that urine is drained before arrival at the site of injury. Ureteroureteral anastomosis should be done only if reimplantation into the bladder is not feasible. Implanting a severed ureter into the bladder is the procedure of choice.

71. The answer is B (1, 3). *(Te Linde, ed 4. p 335.)* Rupture of an interstitial tubal pregnancy can cause severe blood loss, because this area is supplied by both uterine and ovarian vessels. Serious shock usually ensues rapidly. Because interstitial tubal pregnancies usually rupture at a later stage than other tubal pregnancies, a significant percentage can be diagnosed before rupture. Women who have had salpingectomies are at increased risk for interstitial pregnancy.

72. The answer is B (1, 3). *(Te Linde, ed 4. pp 225-226.)* Presacral neurectomy can be an effective therapy both for women who have primary or secondary dysmenorrhea that is unresponsive to medical management and for women who have endometriosis that can be surgically excised without removal of the uterus. Presacral neurectomy does not provide adequate relief from pain secondary to pelvic carcinoma; a better treatment is for a neurosurgeon to sever the nerve fiber near the spinal cord. Because dyspareunia, in the absence of an organic cause, is usually psychic in origin, presacral neurectomy is of little or no benefit.

73. The answer is E (all). *(Te Linde, ed 4. pp 366-369.)* Pregnancy and appendicitis share many of the same signs and symptoms, including nausea, vomiting, abdominal discomfort, constipation, and leukocytosis. Because urinary-tract symptoms are associated commonly with appendicitis of pregnant women, the disease also can be mistaken for pyelitis. Rates of maternal mortality and fetal prematurity are increased in women who are pregnant and have appendicitis.

74-77. The answers are: 74-E, 75-D, 76-C, 77-B. *(Behrman, ed 2. pp 224-225.)* Salpingolysis, salpingoplasty, and uterotubal implantation are the major surgical techniques utilized by tubal surgeons. A salpingolysis is merely the cutting of adhesions surrounding the uterine tube. Salpingoplasty, which is performed on the fimbriated end of the tube, is divided into two parts: fimbriolysis, which is a simple cutting of adhesions causing the fimbria to conglutinate in the midline, and salpingostomy, which is creation of an opening in tubes that were completely closed with hydrosalpinx, usually secondary to infection. On occasion, the tube is occluded at the cornual area, which must be excised and a new opening into the uterus created; this procedure is uterotubal implantation.

Gynecology
Sexuality

John F. Steege

DIRECTIONS: Each question below contains five suggested answers. Choose the **one best** response to each question.

78. All of the following phases of the sex response cycle, as described by Masters and Johnson, are present in both men and women EXCEPT

(A) resolution phase
(B) excitement phase
(C) orgasmic phase
(D) refractory period
(E) plateau phase

79. Penile erection occurs early in the excitement phase of male sexual response. The physiologic action most likely to occur during the same phase of female sexual response is

(A) secretion from Bartholin's glands
(B) lubrication of the vaginal walls
(C) erection of the clitoral shaft
(D) tumescence of the clitoral glans
(E) engorgement of the labia minora

80. According to Masters and Johnson, factors that increase the likelihood of female orgasm during intercourse include

(A) a larger clitoral glans
(B) a clitoris located closer to the vaginal introitus
(C) erection of the clitoral shaft
(D) male superior coital position
(E) none of the above

81. Aspects of female sexual response that have been shown to actively promote fertilization include

(A) dilatation of the cervical os during resolution phase
(B) development of an "orgasmic platform" in the outer third of the vagina
(C) a "sucking" motion due to uterine contractions in orgasm
(D) retreat of the uterus during resolution phase from its elevated position during orgasm
(E) none of the above

82. After having intercourse for several minutes, a woman reaches plateau phase; but she becomes worried when she notices that her partner's penis doesn't seem as large as it did when intercourse began. She is most likely noticing the effect of

(A) lateral retraction of the labia majora and minora
(B) increasing amounts of vaginal lubrication
(C) "tenting" of the upper two-thirds of the vagina
(D) a decrease in vaginal sensitivity that sometimes precedes formation of the "orgasmic platform"
(E) her partner's loss of his erection

83. In the experience of Masters and Johnson and other sex therapists, the sexual dysfunction having the lowest cure rate is

(A) premature ejaculation
(B) vaginismus
(C) primary impotence
(D) secondary impotence
(E) female orgasmic dysfunction

84. The external genitalia of a human embryo begin to clearly differentiate into male or female structures by

(A) 5 weeks gestation
(B) 8 weeks gestation
(C) 10 weeks gestation
(D) 12 weeks gestation
(E) 14 weeks gestation

DIRECTIONS: Each question below contains four suggested answers of which **one** or **more** is correct. Choose the answer:

A	if	**1, 2, and 3**	are correct
B	if	**1 and 3**	are correct
C	if	**2 and 4**	are correct
D	if	**4**	is correct
E	if	**1, 2, 3, and 4**	are correct

85. Masters and Johnson interviewed 331 women concerning their attitudes toward sexual activity during menstruation. This study revealed that

(1) approximately 20 percent of these women objected to it on aesthetic grounds
(2) approximately 50 percent of these women were positively interested in it
(3) approximately 20 percent of these women objected to it on religious grounds
(4) many women's attitudes were affected by the opinions of their male partners

86. Coitus interruptus (withdrawal) often fails as a method of birth control, because

(1) prostatic secretions containing sperm are released during the excitement and plateau phases of sex response
(2) pelvic thrusting becomes involuntary before ejaculation occurs
(3) many men start ejaculating before they realize it
(4) Cowper's gland secretions often contain sperm

87. Extragenital responses during orgasm often include which of the following?

(1) Tachycardia
(2) Sex flush
(3) Elevated blood pressure
(4) Erection of the nipples

88. Significant components of vaginal lubrication include

(1) fluid from Skene's glands
(2) mucus produced by endocervical glands
(3) viscous fluid from Bartholin's glands
(4) transudate-like material from the vaginal walls

89. Although the incidence of rape is increasing in the United States, data indicate that three out of every four rapes still are not reported to law enforcement authorities. Which of the following statements about rape are true?

(1) Rape usually results in pregnancy
(2) Many rapes are perpetrated by men who find violence necessary for sexual fulfillment
(3) Tests for venereal disease should not be performed on rape victims immediately following a rape
(4) Rape can cause sexual dysfunction

90. According to Masters and Johnson, which of the following statements concerning elevation of the uterus during the plateau phase of the female sexual cycle are true?

(1) It may be due to a shortening of the round and uterosacral ligaments
(2) It may be due to vascular congestion in the broad ligaments
(3) It does not occur if the uterus is retroverted
(4) In early plateau, it may be due to negative intra-abdominal pressure caused by hyperventilation

91. Although women's reactions to pregnancy vary, certain physiologic and psychologic changes in sexuality are very common. These include

(1) greater narrowing of the vaginal introitus in the plateau phase
(2) a slower decrease in pelvic vascular congestion during the resolution phase
(3) uncomfortable breast tenderness during sexual stimulation in the first trimester
(4) higher levels of sexual interest and response during the second trimester compared to other times in pregnancy

92. In postmenopausal women, which of the following changes in sexual response are frequently observed?

(1) The upper two-thirds of the vagina expands less during the plateau phase
(2) Uterine contractions during orgasm are frequently more painful
(3) The "sex flush" appears much less commonly
(4) Nipple erection ceases

93. A man and a woman, both 70 years old, consult a sex therapist because of the man's impotence. The woman first became concerned when he failed to ejaculate on several occasions and the man finally agreed that therapy was needed when his erections disappeared completely (except for occasional erections upon awaking). The therapist should tell the couple that

(1) the man's morning erections are not an indication that his physiologic sexual response is intact
(2) older men frequently experience orgasm without ejaculation
(3) the loss of the ability to have an erection is a normal consequence of the aging process
(4) ejaculatory demand decreases with age

SUMMARY OF DIRECTIONS

A	B	C	D	E
1, 2, 3 only	1, 3 only	2, 4 only	4 only	All are correct

94. Which of the following statements describe the syndrome of vaginismus?

(1) It involves involuntary reflex contraction of pelvic perineal and vaginal musculature
(2) It usually is not associated with concomitant dysfunction in the male partner
(3) Affected women can be helped by counseling and the use of vaginal dilators
(4) Diagnosis can be definitely established by history

95. Because it is a systemic disease that can affect vascular and neurologic function, diabetes often alters sexual performance. Problems commonly encountered by diabetic individuals include

(1) frequent vaginal infections
(2) simultaneous onset of impotence and decrease of libido in men
(3) loss of previously established orgasmic capacity in women
(4) loss of uterine and vaginal contractions during orgasmic response

96. Which of the following statements about sexual activity in late pregnancy are true?

(1) Intercourse during the third trimester can lead to premature labor
(2) Intercourse during the third trimester can promote premature rupture of membranes and intrauterine infection
(3) Prostaglandins in semen have been shown to contribute to the initiation of labor
(4) Orgasm is contraindicated in women who have a history of premature labor

97. In recent years there have been several reports ranging from scientific studies to popular books (such as *The Hite Report*) written about women's responses to sexual stimuli. Which of the following statements are supported by these reports?

(1) Vaginal stimulation is as important as clitoral stimulation in achieving orgasm
(2) Direct manipulation of the clitoral glans is often a successful method of achieving orgasm
(3) Most women experience little variation in the intensity and duration of their orgasms
(4) Some women can achieve orgasm without any form of genital stimulation

98. Drugs that have a proven and direct association with either impotence in men or lack of vaginal lubrication in women include which of the following?

(1) Marihuana
(2) Guanethidine (Ismelin)
(3) Hydralazine (Apresoline)
(4) Alpha-methyldopa (Aldomet)

99. Which of the following statements about primary orgasmic dysfunction in women are true?

(1) It can stem from dissatisfaction with a partner's behavior patterns
(2) The influence of orthodox religious beliefs is still of major etiologic significance
(3) It can be exacerbated if the sexual partner suffers from premature ejaculation
(4) An affected woman has never achieved orgasm in her life

100. Female dyspareunia can be described by which of the following statements?

(1) It rarely affects postmenopausal women
(2) Complaints of pain during penile thrusting typically indicate pelvic pathology
(3) Bacterial vaginal infection is a minor etiologic factor
(4) It can develop from sensitivity to intravaginal contraceptive agents

101. Which of the following physiologic actions occur during the plateau phase of sexual excitement in women?

(1) Areolar tumescence
(2) Systolic blood pressure elevations
(3) Involuntary skeletal muscle contractions
(4) Involuntary contractions of the rectal sphincter

Gynecology
Sexuality

Answers

78. The answer is D. *(Masters, 1966. pp 4-7, 13.)* Masters and Johnson observed sexual response in 382 women and 312 men. They arbitrarily divided the sex response cycle of women into the excitement phase, the plateau phase, the orgasmic phase, and the resolution phase. After orgasm, men must wait until a "refractory period" has passed in order for effective restimulation to be possible. The length of this refractory period increases with age.

79. The answer is B. *(Masters, 1966. pp 40, 43-44, 48.)* A woman's initial pelvic response to sexual stimulation is the production of vaginal lubrication, which occurs early in the excitement phase. Considerably later in the same phase, the clitoral glans may increase in diameter. Only if direct manipulation of the clitoris is carried out will the shaft of the clitoris elongate. The labia engorge during late excitement phase, and Bartholin's glands become active in late excitement phase and early plateau phase.

80. The answer is E. *(Dickinson, p 46. Dickinson, JAMA 85[1925]: 1113-1117. Masters, 1966. pp 48, 56-59.)* Masters and Johnson have shown that the size of the clitoris bears no relation to increased orgasmic capacity. Similarly, the distance between the clitoris and the vaginal introitus makes little difference, because clitoral stimulation during coition is provided largely by traction on the clitoral hood via the labia minora, which are moved during penile thrusting. Direct clitoral stimulation can be achieved only by the lateral and female superior coital positions. Erection of the clitoris is likewise not related to orgasmic capacity. Masters and Johnson's findings agree with those of earlier researchers, including Dickinson and Pierson.

81. The answer is E. *(Masters, 1966. pp 115-116, 123-124.)* None of the choices mentioned in the question have been shown to have an active role in enhancing fertility. By placing radiopaque fluid behind cervical caps in six women and taking x-rays during different stages of the sexual response cycle, Masters and Johnson demonstrated that, because no contrast material was drawn up into the uterus, the supposed "sucking" action of the uterus cannot aid in sperm migration. Uterine descent into the seminal pool also is not likely to be important, because the capacity for orgasm has never been correlated with fertility. Cervical gaping may have a minor, passive role in increasing spermatozoal access to the uterine cavity.

82. The answer is C. *(Masters, 1966. pp 39, 76-77, 194.)* During plateau the upper two-thirds of the vagina may suddenly expand further in its transverse and longitudinal dimensions, leading a woman to feel that her vagina is suddenly less full. She may mistakenly assume that her partner's erection has decreased. Lateral retraction of the labia is an earlier event and does not lessen sensation. Similarly, the outer third of the vagina, which engorges with blood to form the "orgasmic platform" in late plateau phase, does not lose its sensitivity.

83. The answer is C. *(Masters, 1970. p 367.)* In a five-year follow-up study of couples treated by Masters and Johnson, the cure rates for vaginismus and premature ejaculation approached 100 percent. Female orgasmic dysfunction was corrected in 80 percent of women, and secondary impotence (impotence despite a history of previous coital success) resolved in 70 percent of men. Primary impotence (chronic and complete inability to maintain an erection sufficient for coitus) was cured only 60 percent of the time. Other therapists report very similar statistics.

84. The answer is B. *(Patten, ed 3. pp 493-499.)* Until about seven weeks gestation, embryonic genitalia are not clearly distinguishable as male or female. After this time, the genital tubercle begins transformation into the clitoris (female) or the glans (male); the genital folds become the labia minora or fuse as the urethral raphe; and the genital swellings develop into the labia majora or the scrotum.

85. The answer is C (2, 4). *(Masters; 1966. pp 125-126.)* Masters and Johnson interviewed 331 women concerning their attitudes toward sexual activity during menstruation. Of these women, approximately 10 percent objected to sexual activity at this time based on religious and aesthetic considerations. Approximately 50 percent of the women were positively interested in sexual activity, especially during the latter half of menstruation, and the remaining women were essentially indifferent provided that they felt well, were not menstruating extremely heavily, and felt there were no aesthetic objections from their male partners. Approximately 13 percent of the women felt that sexual activity decreased dysmenorrhea, and Masters and Johnson clinically demonstrated that sexual activity during menstruation in fact caused a uterine contractile response and temporarily increased the rate of menstrual flow.

86. The answer is C (2, 4). *(Masters, 1966. pp 293, 298.)* Cowper's gland secretions, released in late plateau phase, are thought to contain sperm. Prostatic secretions probably do not contribute to this pre-ejaculatory emission. At the very end of the plateau phase, voluntary pelvic thrusting can become involuntary, therefore making withdrawal of the penis difficult. For two or three seconds before ejaculation, prostatic secretions fill the prostatic urethra, resulting in a feeling that the ejaculation is coming ("ejaculatory inevitability").

87. The answer is B (1, 3). *(Masters, 1966. pp 30-36, 171-176.)* Masters and Johnson documented rises in pulse rate (up to 180 per minute) and blood pressure (systolic elevations of 30 to 80 mm Hg and diastolic elevations of 20 to 40 mm Hg in women). Nipple erection is a late excitement-phase response for men and women, and the "sex flush," a measles-like rash over the chest, abdomen, forearms, and legs, occurs in late plateau in about 75 percent of women and 50 percent of men. (Vital-sign changes measured by Masters and Johnson may have been affected by the laboratory environment.)

88. The answer is D (4). *(Masters, 1966. p 69.)* Masters and Johnson observed a transudate-like fluid emanating directly from the vaginal walls during sexual response. This mucoid material, which is sufficient for complete vaginal lubrication, is produced by transudation from the venous plexus surrounding the vagina and appears seconds after the initiation of sexual excitement. No Skene's gland activity was noted, and production of cervical mucus during sexual stimulation was observed in only a very few subjects. Fluid from Bartholin's glands appears long after vaginal lubrication is well established; it may, however, make a minor contribution to lubrication in late plateau phase.

89. The answer is C (2, 4). *(American Medical Association Committee on Human Sexuality, pp 138-139.)* Although rape does not usually cause pregnancy, it can result in numerous emotional and physical sequelae, including sexual dysfunction, venereal disease, hatred and fear of men, and feelings of guilt. A physician's responsibility to a rape victim is to make sure she is protected prophylactically against pregnancy, to carefully record medical evidence of the rape, and to provide for counseling. Although tests for venereal disease immediately following a rape could not yet be positive as a result of the rape and although the testing itself can be emotionally harmful, for medicolegal reasons these tests should be performed immediately to document absence of disease in the victim at the time of the rape. In one study of sexual offenders, the most common type of offender was men who randomly selected unknown victims and found violence to be necessary for sexual fulfillment.

90. The answer is A (1, 2, 3). *(Masters, 1966. pp 112-114.)* By performing bimanual pelvic examinations during female sexual-response cycles, Masters and Johnson determined that the uterus, unless retroverted, elevates higher into the pelvis in late plateau phase. They hypothesized that vascular congestion of the broad ligaments or shortening of the round and uterosacral ligaments (or both) could cause this phenomenon. Negative intra-abdominal pressure may contribute to elevation of the uterus when hyperventilation occurs in very late plateau phase, but it does not account for elevation earlier in plateau.

91. The answer is E (all). *(Masters, 1966. pp 143-150, 156-160.)* Masters and Johnson demonstrated that pregnant women, compared to nonpregnant women, have a greater narrowing of the vaginal introitus during the plateau phase and a slower decrease in pelvic vascular congestion in the resolution phase. In addition, breasts are especially tender to sexual stimulation in the first trimester, particularly among nulliparous women; and sexual interest and response increase in the second trimester. Masters and Johnson attributed these phenomena to the hypervolemic state of pregnancy, which seems to accentuate vascular congestion changes of the sexual response cycle.

92. The answer is A (1,2,3). *(Masters, 1966. pp 224, 227, 233, 237.)* After menopause, vaginal walls become thinner, lose their rugae, and become less elastic. As a result, vaginal expansion in plateau phase is reduced. Peripheral neurovascular response (the sex flush) rarely appears in postmenopausal women, probably as a result of estrogen deprivation. Similarly, uterine contractions, which normally proceed in premenopausal women in coordinated fashion from fundus to lower uterine segment, may become irregular and spastic with age, resulting in uncomfortable cramps. These symptoms are relieved by estrogen replacement. Nipple erection is not affected by senescence, although breast engorgement diminishes with age, especially if a woman has breast-fed babies in the past.

93. The answer is D (4). *(Masters, 1970. pp 322-325.)* The presence of morning erections indicates adequate physiologic sexual capacity and remains the best historical guide for screening men complaining of impotence. The capacity for erection generally persists into old age, unless directly interfered with by medications or medical illness. More lengthy and direct genital stimulation may be needed for an older man to attain full erection. The feeling of a need to ejaculate ("ejaculatory demand") decreases with age. If one or both sexual partners feel that coitus is incomplete without ejaculation or that a man is harmed by not ejaculating, feelings of inadequacy can develop, leading ultimately to impotence. Orgasm is almost invariably accompanied by ejaculation.

94. The answer is B (1, 3). *(Masters, 1970. pp 250-251, 262-265.)* Vaginismus is defined as the involuntary spastic contraction of the pelvic musculature of the perineum and outer one-third of the vagina. Although a history of vaginal "tightness" or pain on entry is highly suggestive of vaginismus, the diagnosis must be verified by demonstrating involuntary spasm on pelvic examination. A large proportion of partners of women who have vaginismus have primary or secondary impotence. Counseling and the use of vaginal dilators can be highly successful in treating women affected by vaginismus.

95. The answer is B (1, 3). *(Ellenberg, Ann Intern Med 75[1971]:213-219. Kolodny, Diabetes 20[1971]: 557-559. Lief, pp 117-118.)* Susceptibility of diabetic women to fungal and bacterial vaginitis, which can cause irritation during coitus, may be a contributing factor in the disappearance of orgasmic response, which occurs in about 30 percent of women who have diabetes. Neurologic factors, however, have not been adequately explored. There is no evidence that orgasm, when it does occur, differs between diabetic and nondiabetic women. Men who have diabetes may notice diminished erectile capacity as much as a year before diabetes becomes clinically evident. Libido generally remains unimpaired.

96. The answer is D (4). *(Green, pp 133-144.)* Several clinical surveys have failed to reveal any firm association between intercourse and premature labor, premature rupture of membranes, or intrauterine infection. On the other hand, orgasm, regardless of how it is achieved, can be harmful to women who have a history of premature delivery or a prematurely ripe cervix, because of accompanying uterine contractions. A fetal head that is engaged in the pelvis may be bumped during coitus; although this may frighten the parents, no demonstrable harm to the infant results. The physiologic role of prostaglandins in human semen is unknown.

97. The answer is D (4). *(Masters, 1966. pp 63, 67. Romney, pp 528-529.)* Although most women state that they are sexually stimulated by both vaginal and clitoral sensations, less than 10 percent feel that vaginal sensation is the more significant. In fact, regardless of the various sources of sexual stimulation, orgasm is in the vast majority of cases achieved through clitoral stimulation. However, in rare cases, women have achieved scientifically documented orgasms through breast stimulation alone. Women usually find stimulation of the mons or the clitoral shaft more pleasing than direct stimulation of the clitoral glans, which is an extremely sensitive organ. The duration and intensity of orgasm varies greatly from woman to woman and from one experience to another.

98. The answer is D (4). *(Alderman, N Engl J Med 293[1975]: 65-68. Bock, Ger Med Mon 13[1968]: 449-450. Goodman, ed 5. p 556. Kolodny, pp 18-22. Lief, pp 309-310. Pillay, S Afr Med J 50[1976]: 625-626.)* Although marihuana is felt by many to enhance their experiences of orgasm, because it can alter time perception, effects on erection or vaginal lubrication have not been reported. Guanethidine (Ismelin), an adrenergic-neuron blocking agent, is sympatholytic and thus can inhibit ejaculation; impotence then can develop for psychogenic reasons. It is not known if loss of orgasmic response occurs in women taking guanethidine. Alpha-methyldopa (Aldomet) produced impotence in 15 to at least 35 percent of men in various clinical series, depending somewhat on the dose. Hydralazine (Apresoline) may inhibit erection in about 15 percent of men, but proof of this effect is lacking. Similarly, the possible effects of alpha-methyldopa and hydralazine on vaginal lubrication warrant further clinical investigation.

99. The answer is E (all). *(Masters, 1970. pp 227-237.)* Many factors can contribute to the development of primary orgasmic dysfunction in women. By definition, these women have not been able to achieve orgasm through any physical means at any time in their lives; reasons for their dysfunction can include the influence of traditional orthodox religious beliefs, dissatisfaction with their partners' behavioral or social traits, past trauma (such as rape), or rigid familial sexual proscriptions. Sexual dysfunction, particularly premature ejaculation, in a male partner can reinforce a woman's orgasmic dysfunction.

100. The answer is D (4). *(Masters, 1970. pp 266-288.)* Aside from psychological causes, female dyspareunia also can stem from a number of physical disorders. Infection of the vaginal barrel, such as with *Escherichia coli* or *Streptococcus faecalis*, can cause distressful burning and aching during and after coition. Insufficient vaginal lubrication also can cause dyspareunia; this condition can occur in postmenopausal women who are not receiving estrogen replacement therapy. Sensitivity to intravaginal chemical contraceptives and irritation of the clitoris, vaginal outlet, or labia can lead to dyspareunia. A woman's complaint of pain during penile thrusting is difficult to evaluate; although this pain can indicate pelvic disorders, such as laceration of uterine ligaments, it also frequently stems from a desire to avoid intercourse.

101. The answer is A (1, 2, 3). *(Masters, 1966. pp 27-37.)* The response of women to sexual stimulation is generalized and affects many different organ systems. Physiologic responses include superficial and deep vasocongestion accounting for, among other things, enlargement and changes of color of extragenital and genital areas. Voluntary and involuntary myotonia, both generalized and specific, also may occur, although involuntary contractions of the rectal sphincter are usually detected only during the orgasmic phase.

Oncology

Peter E. Schwartz
Barney B. Silverman

DIRECTIONS: Each question below contains five suggested answers. Choose the **one best** response to each question.

102. A 19-year-old Taiwanese woman is expecting her first child; she is 12 weeks pregnant by dates. She has vaginal bleeding and a uterus of proportions found at 20 weeks gestation. A sample of tissue she has passed vaginally is shown below. The most likely diagnosis is

(A) sarcoma botryoides
(B) tuberculous endometritis
(C) adenocarcinoma of the uterus
(D) hydatidiform mole
(E) normal pregnancy

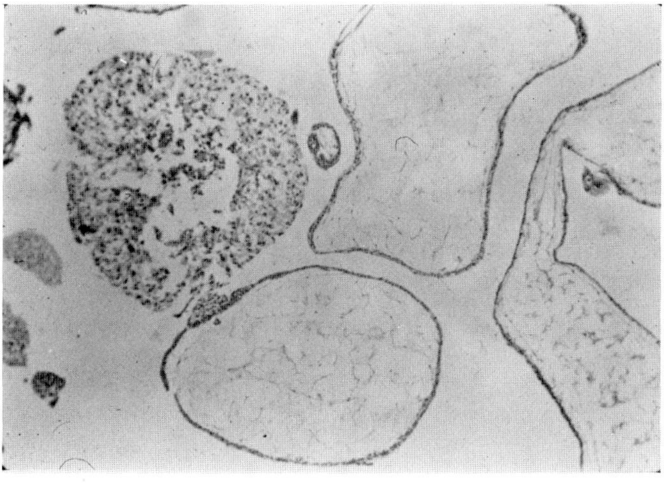

103. Young women whose mothers took diethylstilbestrol during pregnancy are most likely to develop which of the following vaginal carcinomas?

(A) Papillary adenocarcinoma
(B) Squamous carcinoma
(C) Carcinoma of the infantile vagina
(D) Adenosquamous carcinoma
(E) Clear cell adenocarcinoma

104. Which of the following statements about carcinoma of the vagina is true?

(A) It most commonly occurs in the lateral walls of the lower one-third of the vagina
(B) Its incidence is highest in women in their fifties and sixties
(C) It is rarely epidermoid
(D) Most affected women have adenocarcinoma
(E) Primary malignancies are more common than secondary malignancies

105. A 71-year-old woman has postmenopausal bleeding. Fractional dilatation and curettage reveals adenocarcinoma confined to the endometrium. The most important prognostic factor for this woman would be

(A) her age
(B) the tumor grade
(C) the size of her uterus
(D) the depth of myometrial invasion
(E) none of the above

106. Fractional dilatation and curettage reveals endometrial carcinoma involving the cervix. This finding is

(A) of no prognostic significance
(B) of minor prognostic significance but does not require change in management
(C) significant only if the cervical tumor is clinically obvious
(D) significant even if the disease is present only microscopically
(E) contraindicative for hysterectomy

107. The primary mode of treatment for endometrial carcinoma confined to the uterine corpus is

(A) external beam radiation
(B) intracavitary radium
(C) hysterectomy
(D) chemotherapy
(E) progestin therapy

108. Women who have endometrial carcinoma most frequently present with which of the following symptoms?

(A) Bloating
(B) Weight loss
(C) Postmenopausal bleeding
(D) Vaginal discharge
(E) Hemoptysis

109. The exogenous factor most often associated with the development of anaplastic endometrial carcinoma and mixed mesodermal tumor of the uterus is

(A) ingestion of conjugated estrogens
(B) ingestion of sequential birth-control pills
(C) ingestion of combined birth-control pills
(D) prior pelvic irradiation
(E) placement of an intrauterine contraceptive device

110. For postmenopausal women in whom cystic glandular hyperplasia of the endometrium has been diagnosed by fractional dilatation and curettage, the usual management is

(A) hysterectomy
(B) hysterectomy preceded by radiation
(C) hysterectomy followed by radiation
(D) hysterectomy and bilateral salpingo-oophorectomy
(E) observation

111. The class of chemotherapeutic agents that is most effective in the management of patients who have recurrent endometrial carcinoma is

(A) antimetabolites
(B) hormones
(C) alkylating agents
(D) vinca alkaloids
(E) antibiotics

112. The most common sarcoma of the uterus is

(A) leiomyosarcoma
(B) rhabdomyosarcoma
(C) endometrial stromal sarcoma
(D) carcinosarcoma
(E) mixed mesodermal sarcoma

113. Metastatic adenocarcinoma of the uterus develops most commonly from cancer of the

(A) ovary
(B) stomach
(C) breast
(D) fallopian tube
(E) vagina

114. Adenoacanthoma of the uterus is considered to represent

(A) a combination malignancy from two separate sources
(B) an adenocarcinoma with squamous metaplasia
(C) an extension of extrauterine adenoacanthoma
(D) a neoplastic transformation of "indifferent" cells beneath normal uterine epithelium
(E) none of the above

115. Ovarian neoplasms most commonly arise from

(A) coelomic epithelium
(B) nonspecific mesenchyme
(C) specialized gonadal stroma
(D) primitive germ cells
(E) none of the above

116. Mixed mesodermal tumors of the uterus can be described by which of the following statements?

(A) They are more common than previously assumed and comprise about 17 to 18 percent of uterine malignancies
(B) Microscopic examination may reveal the presence of bone, cartilage, muscle, or other elements
(C) Their development has been associated with maternal intake of estrogen during pregnancy
(D) Five-year survival rate is quite good (approximately 80 percent)
(E) They are not known to occur before the menopausal years

117. A 25-year-old woman complains of diarrhea and weight loss; her heart rate is 130 per minute. Head, neck, and chest x-rays, upper gastrointestinal series, small-bowel followthrough, and barium enema all are negative. An ovarian lesion, discovered during laparotomy, is biopsied (a photomicrograph of a specimen is shown below) and excised. After her tumor was removed, the woman's symptoms disappeared. The most likely diagnosis is

(A) carcinoid tumor
(B) endometriosis
(C) struma ovarii
(D) embryonal teratoma
(E) dysgerminoma

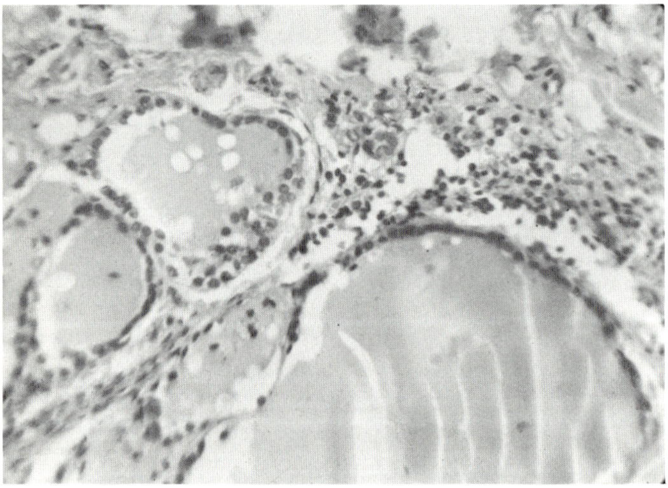

118. All of the following statements regarding ovarian cancer are true EXCEPT

(A) it is the most common gynecologic cancer
(B) it has the highest mortality rate among the common gynecologic cancers
(C) it tends to be asymptomatic until it has reached an advanced stage
(D) its development may be influenced by environmental, cultural, or socioeconomic factors
(E) Pap smears are ineffective for routine diagnostic screening

119. Which of the following groups of chemotherapeutic agents has been most effective in treating women who have ovarian epithelial tumors?

(A) Antimetabolites
(B) Hormones
(C) Alkylating agents
(D) Vinca alkaloids
(E) Antibiotics

120. Women who have ovarian carcinoma most commonly present with which of the following symptoms?

(A) Vaginal bleeding and anorexia
(B) Weight loss and dyspareunia
(C) Nausea and vaginal discharge
(D) Constipation and frequent urination
(E) Abdominal distension and pain

121. Which of the following statements about the International Federation of Gynecology and Obstetrics (FIGO) staging of ovarian carcinoma is true?

(A) Stages I through VI have been defined
(B) Stage II carcinoma is limited to the ovaries
(C) The presence of ascites is significant in differentiating between substages of Stage III
(D) Ovarian involvement and spread outside the peritoneal cavity characterize Stage IV
(E) The FIGO grouping is based on clinical examination only

122. Pelvic examination of a 19-year-old woman who complains of lower abdominal discomfort reveals a mobile, six-centimeter mass in the anterior cul-de-sac. The most likely diagnosis is

(A) serous carcinoma
(B) urachal cyst
(C) benign cystic teratoma
(D) intraligamentous fibroid
(E) diverticular abscess

123. The major mode of spread of ovarian neoplasms is by way of

(A) ovarian veins
(B) ovarian vein lymphatics
(C) pelvic lymphatics
(D) local extension
(E) peritoneal seeding

124. All of the following statements about mesonephroid carcinoma of the ovary are true EXCEPT

(A) it occurs less frequently than mucinous carcinoma
(B) it probably arises from embryonic rests of mesonephric origin
(C) it may contain endometrioid areas
(D) it is associated with pelvic endometriosis more often than endometrioid carcinoma
(E) five-year survival rate of affected women approaches 50 percent

125. Which of the following statements about Brenner tumors of the ovary is NOT true?

(A) They generally are benign
(B) They are characterized microscopically by areas of epithelial cells surrounded by mesenchymal tissue
(C) Their cells have a characteristic "coffee-bean" nucleus
(D) They tend to grow rather slowly
(E) They rarely are larger than 2 cm in diameter

126. The use of intraperitoneal radioisotope therapy is most effective in the treatment of women who have which of the following sequelae of ovarian epithelial carcinoma?

(A) Rupture of malignant ovarian cysts
(B) Peritoneal carcinomatosis
(C) Metastasis beyond the abdominal cavity
(D) Omental metastases
(E) Lymphatic spread

127. A 54-year-old woman undergoes a laparotomy because of a pelvic mass, which proves to be a unilateral ovarian neoplasm accompanied by a large omental metastasis. The most appropriate intraoperative course of action would be

(A) omental biopsy
(B) ovarian biopsy
(C) excision of the omental metastasis and unilateral oophorectomy
(D) omentectomy and bilateral salpingo-oophorectomy
(E) omentectomy, total abdominal hysterectomy, and bilateral salpingo-oophorectomy

128. A 45-year-old woman has undergone a total abdominal hysterectomy and bilateral salpingo-oophorectomy for Stage II serous carcinoma of the ovary. The most effective postoperative radiotherapeutic treatment of this woman would be

(A) whole-abdomen irradiation
(B) pelvic irradiation
(C) whole-abdomen and pelvic irradiation
(D) vaginal radium insertion and pelvic irradiation
(E) intraperitoneal radioisotope therapy

129. Women who have clear cell adenocarcinoma of the vagina most frequently present with which of the following symptoms?

(A) Primary amenorrhea
(B) Irregular vaginal bleeding
(C) Pelvic and abdominal masses
(D) Hematuria
(E) Weight loss

130. Which of the following statements in NOT true regarding the use of alkylating agents in the treatment of women who have ovarian cancer?

(A) No agent is best in producing objective responses
(B) No particular schedule of administration is superior
(C) Prior radiation therapy decreases response rates to alkylating agents
(D) Intraperitoneal administration is as effective as systemic administration
(E) Toxicity, but not response, is enhanced by intense, high-dose intravenous treatment

131. Routine pelvic examination reveals that a 21-year-old woman has a hooded cervix. This finding is most frequently associated with

(A) pregnancy
(B) traumatic abortion
(C) in utero drug exposure
(D) a prior Shirodkar procedure
(E) a herpes infection

132. The majority of deaths from cervical carcinoma can be attributed to

(A) local extension
(B) metastasis to the central nervous system
(C) metastasis to the liver and lungs
(D) iatrogenic causes
(E) none of the above

133. Carcinoma in situ of the cervix is characterized by all of the following EXCEPT

(A) involvement of the entire thickness of the squamous epithelium
(B) cells resembling those of invasive carcinoma
(C) evidence of stromal invasion
(D) complete loss of stratification
(E) occasional regression and disappearance

134. Stage IIb carcinoma of the cervix is defined by

(A) involvement only of the cervix with early stromal invasion
(B) extension to the corpus uteri without parametrial involvement
(C) extension beyond the cervix (but not to the pelvic wall or the lower one-third of the vagina) without obvious parametrial involvement
(D) extension beyond the cervix (but not to the pelvic wall or the lower one-third of the vagina) with obvious parametrial involvement
(E) extension to the pelvic wall and involvement of the upper one-third of the vagina

135. Secondary involvement with cervical carcinoma most frequently occurs in the

(A) corpus uteri
(B) portio vaginalis
(C) parametrium
(D) uterosacral ligaments
(E) external inguinal lymph nodes

136. The cervical neoplastic disease most likely to develop in women who were exposed in utero to diethylstilbestrol is

(A) microglandular hyperplasia
(B) squamous cell carcinoma
(C) clear cell adenocarcinoma
(D) papillary adenocarcinoma
(E) none of the above

137. The neoplasm most sensitive to appropriate chemotherapy is

(A) gestational trophoblastic disease
(B) ovarian dysgerminoma
(C) Burkitt's lymphoma
(D) endometrial carcinoma
(E) ovarian serous carcinoma

138. A 23-year-old primigravid woman undergoes spontaneous evacuation of a hydatidiform mole; a completion curettage subsequently confirms the diagnosis. The patient has no clinical or radiographic evidence of metastatic disease. Management of this woman should include

(A) weekly human chorionic gonadotropin (HCG) titers
(B) hysterectomy
(C) single-agent chemotherapy
(D) combination chemotherapy
(E) radiation therapy

139. The presence of adnexal masses in a woman who has a hydatidiform mole is an indication for

(A) hormone therapy
(B) radiation therapy
(C) emergency surgical intervention
(D) eventual surgical intervention
(E) none of the above

140. A 17-year-old primigravid woman, during the twelfth week of her pregnancy, has vaginal bleeding and an enlarged-for-dates uterus. In addition, no fetal heart tones are heard. The safest and most reliable method for early diagnosis of hydatidiform mole, prior to spontaneous evacuation, is

(A) amniography
(B) ultrasonography
(C) plain film of the abdomen
(D) pelvic arteriography
(E) HCG titer

141. Which of the following would be the most effective means of determining the presence of a growing tumor in a patient who has gestational trophoblastic disease?

(A) Serial chest x-rays
(B) Size of adnexal masses
(C) Evaluation of menstrual function
(D) Presence of lactation
(E) Serial HCG titers

142. Extramammary Paget's disease of the vulva is associated with which of the following cancers?

(A) Melanoma
(B) Leiomyosarcoma
(C) Squamous carcinoma
(D) Apocrine gland carcinoma
(E) Bartholin's gland carcinoma

143. A 55-year-old woman has a three-centimeter raised irregular white lesion at the mucocutaneous junction of the vulva. A sample of the biopsied lesion is shown below. The most likely diagnosis is

(A) tuberculosis of the vulva
(B) Bowen's Disease
(C) Paget's Disease
(D) invasive squamous cell carcinoma of the vulva
(E) fibrosarcoma of the vulva

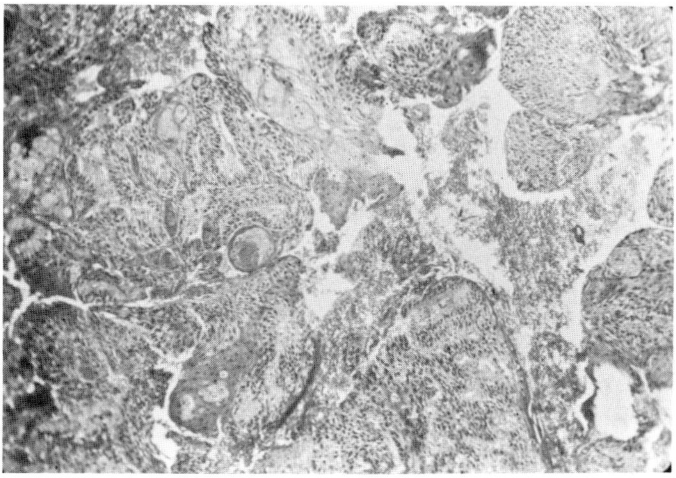

144. A woman is found to have a unilateral, invasive vulvar carcinoma that is 2 cm in diameter but that is not associated with evidence of lymph-node spread. Initial management of this woman most likely would consist of

(A) chemotherapy
(B) radiation therapy
(C) simple vulvectomy
(D) radical vulvectomy
(E) radical vulvectomy and bilateral inguinal lymphadenectomy

DIRECTIONS: Each question below contains four suggested answers of which **one** or **more** is correct. Choose the answer:

A	if	**1, 2, and 3**	are correct
B	if	**1 and 3**	are correct
C	if	**2 and 4**	are correct
D	if	**4**	is correct
E	if	**1, 2, 3, and 4**	are correct

145. Endometrial adenocarcinoma has been associated with

(1) adenomatous hyperplasia
(2) late menopause
(3) estrogen therapy
(4) multiparity

146. Recent evidence in evaluating cell types found in carcinoma of the endometrium suggests that

(1) poorly differentiated adenocarcinomas have a poor prognosis
(2) adenoacanthomas have a poor prognosis
(3) adenosquamous carcinomas have a poor prognosis
(4) adenosquamous tumors occur more often in young women

147. Adenocarcinoma of the endometrium can be described by which of the following statements?

(1) It is primarily a disease of postmenopausal women
(2) The average age of affected women is ten years more than the average age of women who have cervical carcinoma
(3) It has a more favorable prognosis than cervical cancer, with the five-year survival rate approaching 75 percent
(4) It is increasing in frequency relative to carcinoma of the cervix

148. Which of the following statements correctly match stages of endometrial carcinoma with the appropriate survival rates?

(1) Survival rate should exceed 90 percent if the disease is limited to the endometrium
(2) Survival rate should exceed 80 percent if the myometrium is involved superficially
(3) Survival rate is 50 percent if extensive myometrial or cervical involvement has occurred
(4) Survival rate is no higher than 25 percent if extrauterine spread has occurred

149. For the management of women who have endometrial carcinoma, intracavitary radium has been employed routinely in which of the following ways?

(1) As a treatment for women who have ovarian metastases
(2) As a treatment for women who have vaginal apical recurrences
(3) As a treatment for women who have metastases of the pelvic sidewall
(4) As primary therapy for inoperable patients

150. Indications for external beam radiation therapy in the management of women who have uterine malignancies include

(1) enlarged uterus
(2) anaplastic adenocarcinoma
(3) deep myometrial invasion
(4) gross extension to the cervix

151. Carcinoma of the endometrium in women younger than 40 years of age can be associated with which of the following?

(1) Ovarian choriocarcinoma
(2) Stein-Leventhal syndrome
(3) Dysgerminoma
(4) Diethylstilbestrol ingestion

152. Women who have which of the following characteristics are at high risk for endometrial carcinoma?

(1) Hypertension
(2) Diabetes
(3) Obesity
(4) Familial history of endometrial carcinoma

153. Development of endometrial hyperplasia has been associated with

(1) perimenopausal anovulation
(2) prolonged postpartum anovulation
(3) granulosa-theca-cell tumors
(4) Stein-Leventhal syndrome

154. How well a patient responds to progestin therapy for recurrent endometrial carcinoma is influenced by which of the following factors?

(1) Volume of the tumor
(2) Differentiation of the tumor
(3) Sites of metastases
(4) Age of the patient

155. Histologic grading of adenocarcinoma of the uterus can be described by which of the following statements?

(1) In the Broders system, Grade IV is the most malignant type of tumor
(2) In the FIGO Cancer Committee system, grade one is the most malignant type of tumor
(3) Grading is valuable prognostically as well as descriptively
(4) The degree of myometrial invasion is the key to histologic grading

156. The spread of adenocarcinoma of the body of the uterus can be described by which of the following statements?

(1) Distant organs, such as the liver, are frequently involved
(2) Dissemination is chiefly by way of the lymphatics
(3) The tumor resembles cervical carcinoma in its frequency of dissemination
(4) Direct extension is an important route of dissemination

SUMMARY OF DIRECTIONS

A	B	C	D	E
1, 2, 3 only	1, 3 only	2, 4 only	4 only	All are correct

157. Pelvic examination is an important means of diagnosing ovarian malignancies. An ovarian tumor is likely to be malignant if examination reveals that it is

(1) mobile
(2) bilateral
(3) cystic
(4) greater than 10 cm in diameter

158. Routine preoperative evaluation of a patient who has a large, fixed, irregular pelvic mass that is highly suggestive of an ovarian tumor should include which of the following diagnostic procedures?

(1) Chest x-ray
(2) Intravenous pyelography
(3) Barium enema
(4) Liver scan

159. During the appendectomy of a 23-year-old woman, an ovarian tumor is discovered. Which of the following findings at the time of surgery would suggest that the tumor is malignant?

(1) Peritoneal implants
(2) Hemorrhagic ascites
(3) Surface excrescences on the ovary
(4) Adhesion to adjacent organs

160. In a young woman for whom conservation of reproductive function is desired, a unilateral salpingo-oophorectomy for selected ovarian malignancies may be performed, provided that the cancer does not extend grossly beyond the involved ovary. Which of the following intraoperative procedures should be performed at this time to reveal microscopic metastases?

(1) Omental biopsy
(2) Peritoneal cytology
(3) Biopsy of the uninvolved ovary
(4) Examination of the diaphragm

161. Stromo-epithelial neoplasms of the ovary can be of which of the following histologic types?

(1) Serous
(2) Mucinous
(3) Endometrioid
(4) Mesonephroid

162. Epithelial ovarian tumors of low potential malignancy (borderline malignancies) can be described by which of the following statements?

(1) They represent nearly half of all epithelial ovarian tumors
(2) They occasionally are associated with late recurrences and death
(3) They seldom, if ever, metastasize within the peritoneal cavity
(4) They are not associated with destructive infiltration of the ovarian stroma

163. Which of the following statements about serous carcinoma of the ovary are true?

(1) It is the most common epithelial carcinoma of the ovary
(2) It often contains psammoma bodies
(3) It is bilateral in approximately one-third of affected women
(4) It frequently is associated with pelvic endometriosis

164. Which of the following statements about mucinous carcinoma of the ovary are true?

(1) It usually is diagnosed at a less advanced stage than serous carcinoma
(2) It tends to be unilateral
(3) It tends to be well differentiated
(4) Affected patients have a five-year survival rate approaching 50 percent

165. Which of the following statements concerning endometrioid carcinoma of the ovary are true?

(1) It rarely occurs in association with endometrial carcinoma
(2) It commonly arises from ovarian endometriosis
(3) It is associated with a poorer five-year survival rate than serous carcinoma
(4) It often has histologic evidence of squamous metaplasia

166. Important prognostic factors concerning ovarian epithelial carcinoma include

(1) extent of the tumor
(2) volume of the tumor
(3) histologic differentiation of the tumor
(4) presence of ascites

167. The use of external-beam radiation therapy in the management of women who have epithelial ovarian cancer generally is avoided if

(1) ascites is observed
(2) the diameter of residual tumor exceeds 2 cm
(3) metastases are present on the peritoneum covering the kidney
(4) retroperitoneal pelvic metastases are present

168. A woman enters a hospital for an exploratory laparotomy, which reveals the presence of epithelial ovarian cancer. As a result, chemotherapy is begun. Factors that may be of prognostic importance in determining whether this woman will have evidence of disease on a "second look" laparotomy include the

(1) number of courses of chemotherapy
(2) amount of clinically palpable tumor
(3) histologic grade of tumor
(4) histologic type of epithelial tumor

SUMMARY OF DIRECTIONS

A	B	C	D	E
1, 2, 3 only	1, 3 only	2, 4 only	4 only	All are correct

169. Which of the following statements describe carcinoma of the ovary?

(1) It causes more deaths annually than cervical carcinoma
(2) It is the cause of death of more than one percent of all women older than 40 years
(3) Its cystic variety is more common than the solid form
(4) It frequently can be diagnosed by routine cytologic smear

170. Development of adenocarcinoma of the vagina has been associated with in utero exposure to which of the following compounds?

(1) Hexestrol
(2) Ethinylestrenol
(3) Dienestrol
(4) Medroxyprogesterone acetate

171. Which of the following statements concerning carcinoma of the vagina are true?

(1) Squamous carcinoma is the most common type
(2) Carcinoma in situ is often multifocal
(3) Metastasis may occur by way of cervical or vulvar lymphatics
(4) Young women are most often affected

172. Vaginal carcinoma in women whose mothers received diethylstilbestrol during pregnancy can be characterized by which of the following statements?

(1) It is most commonly located in the middle and outer portions of the vagina
(2) It classically occurs in women in their teens and early twenties
(3) Electron microscopy has shown that it is müllerian in origin
(4) It occurs in less than 0.1 percent of women exposed in utero to diethylstilbestrol

173. Cervical carcinoma is considered invasive when there is

(1) a breakthrough of the basement membrane
(2) penetration of the stroma
(3) involvement of the lymphatics
(4) involvement of the endocervical glands

174. Which of the following statements about microinvasive carcinoma of the cervix are true?

(1) Its diagnosis requires the presence of glandular involvement
(2) One to two percent of affected patients eventually succumb to the disease
(3) Its diagnosis requires penetration of the disease deeper than 5 mm beneath the basal layer
(4) If stromal or lymphatic invasion has occurred, extensive therapy is necessary

175. The disease process illustrated in the slide below can affect which of the following?

(1) Breast
(2) Cervix
(3) Vulva
(4) Ovary

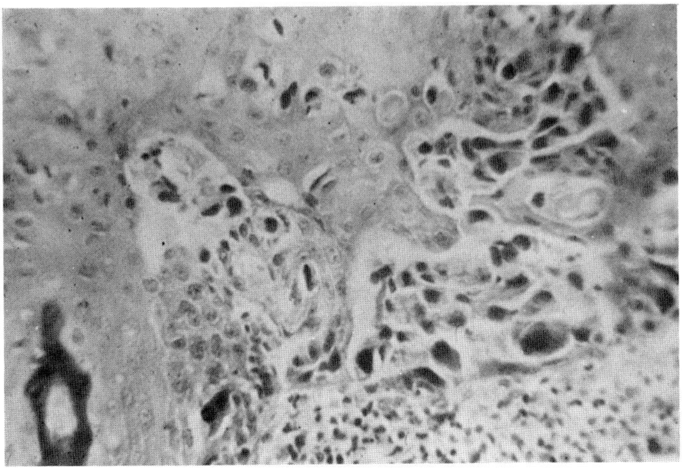

176. Adenocarcinoma of the cervix can be characterized by which of the following statements?

(1) It is more common in older patients than the epidermoid variety
(2) It represents approximately 20 percent of all cervical carcinomas
(3) It usually takes the form of a "clear cell" (mesonephroid) tumor
(4) It characteristically arises within the cervical canal

177. Observations on the role of actinomycin D and methotrexate in the management of gestational trophoblastic disease suggest that

(1) resistance to one agent results in cross-resistance to the other
(2) actinomycin D is safer than methotrexate for women whose liver function is impaired
(3) there is no additive effect in combining the two agents
(4) actinomycin D is as effective as methotrexate for primary treatment

SUMMARY OF DIRECTIONS

A	B	C	D	E
1, 2, 3 only	1, 3 only	2, 4 only	4 only	All are correct

178. A woman who has trophoblastic disease would be considered a high-risk patient if metastases are present in her

(1) brain
(2) lungs
(3) liver
(4) vagina

179. Disorders referred to as "gestational trophoblastic disease" include

(1) hydatidiform mole
(2) chorioadenoma destruens
(3) choriocarcinoma
(4) ovarian choriocarcinoma

180. The histologic classification of gestational trophoblastic disease can be characterized by which of the following statements?

(1) It is a reliable indicator of prognosis
(2) It determines the therapeutic regimen
(3) It defines the probability of complete remission
(4) It is based in part on retention of villus structures

181. Which of the following statements about choriocarcinoma are true?

(1) It usually metastasizes by hematogenous routes
(2) It is preceded by molar pregnancy in about 85 percent of cases
(3) It can occur several years after a molar pregnancy
(4) It most commonly metastasizes to the liver

182. Criteria that are especially reliable in determining a patient's response to chemotherapy for gestational trophoblastic disease include

(1) duration of the disease
(2) urine levels of HCG
(3) sites of metastasis
(4) the patient's age

183. Indications for instituting single-agent chemotherapy following evacuation of a hydatidiform mole usually include

(1) a rise in HCG titers
(2) failure of HCG titers to return to normal four weeks after evacuation
(3) failure of HCG titers to return to normal eight weeks after evacuation
(4) appearance of liver or brain metastases

184. Which of the following statements about carcinoma of the vulva are true?

(1) It usually takes the form of squamous carcinoma
(2) It frequently arises in ducts of Bartholin's gland
(3) It is a disease of older women
(4) It usually is preceded by vulvar dystrophies

185. Primary carcinoma of the vulva can be described by which of the following statements?

(1) It characteristically is preceded by granulomatous disease
(2) It accounts for 3 to 4 percent of all primary genital-canal malignancies
(3) It rarely extends into the stroma
(4) Widespread, distant metastasis is uncommon

186. Factors associated with an increased incidence of regional lymph-node metastasis secondary to carcinoma of the vulva include

(1) tumor size greater than 2 cm
(2) involvement of the anus
(3) involvement of the vagina
(4) extension to the perineum

187. Which of the following statements about epidermoid carcinoma of the vulva are true?

(1) It is associated with an increased incidence of epidermoid carcinoma of the endocervix
(2) It is seen less frequently than adenocarcinoma
(3) It tends to develop in women who are older than those affected by adenocarcinoma
(4) It tends to be more advanced when diagnosed than adenocarcinoma

188. Carcinoma of the fallopian tube can be described by which of the following statements?

(1) It is an uncommon lesion, accounting for approximately 0.2 to 0.5 percent of primary genital-tract malignancies
(2) Bilateral involvement occurs in approximately half of affected patients
(3) Its microscopic appearance can be papillary or papillary-alveolar
(4) It is considered only mildly malignant and is associated with a good five-year survival rate

189. Clinical signs or symptoms frequently associated with carcinoma of the fallopian tube include

(1) vaginal discharge
(2) adnexal mass
(3) abdominal pain
(4) hypermenorrhea

SUMMARY OF DIRECTIONS

A	B	C	D	E
1, 2, 3 only	1, 3 only	2, 4 only	4 only	All are correct

190. Meigs' syndrome can be described by which of the following statements?

(1) Hydrothorax and ascites are the primary features
(2) It rarely is seen in combination with ovarian fibromas
(3) It can occur with Brenner tumor, thecoma, and granulosa cell tumor
(4) It characteristically is associated with large subserous myomas

191. Which of the following statements about ovarian neoplasms in children are true?

(1) They are most often of germ cell origin
(2) They are an infrequent cause of precocious puberty
(3) Coelomic epithelial tumors are usually benign
(4) Tumors of germ cell origin are frequently malignant

192. Which of the following statements about ovarian neoplasms of pregnant women are true?

(1) They are usually malignant
(2) They are most often confined to one ovary
(3) They may spread transplacentally to the fetus
(4) They can be mistaken for a cystic corpus luteum

193. Which of the following statements characterize sarcoma botryoides?

(1) It tends to be multicentric
(2) Its initial manifestation usually is lower abdominal pain
(3) It occurs most frequently in children
(4) Cartilagenous and osseous elements are common

DIRECTIONS: The groups of questions below consist of lettered choices followed by several numbered items. For each numbered item select the **one** lettered choice with which it is **most** closely associated. Each lettered choice may be used once, more than once, or not at all.

Questions 194-198

For each description that follows, select the ovarian tumor with which it is most likely to be associated.

(A) Dysgerminoma
(B) Dermoid cyst
(C) Carcinoid tumor
(D) Embryonal carcinoma
(E) Choriocarcinoma

194. Usually becomes squamous carcinoma when malignant degeneration occurs

195. Most radiosensitive ovarian tumor

196. Can be associated with elevated serum levels of alpha-fetoprotein

197. Routinely treated with combination chemotherapy

198. Often develops in a gonadoblastoma

Questions 199-203

For each description that follows, select the ovarian tumor with which it is most likely to be associated.

(A) Granulosa tumor
(B) Sertoli-Leydig cell tumor
(C) Immature teratoma
(D) Gonadoblastoma
(E) Kruckenberg tumor

199. Frequently associated with virilization

200. Frequently associated with endometrial carcinoma

201. Tends to recur more than five years following the original diagnosis

202. Calcifications present on pelvic radiographs

203. Correlation between malignant potential and the amount of embryogenic tissue

Questions 204-207

Match the following ovarian tumors.

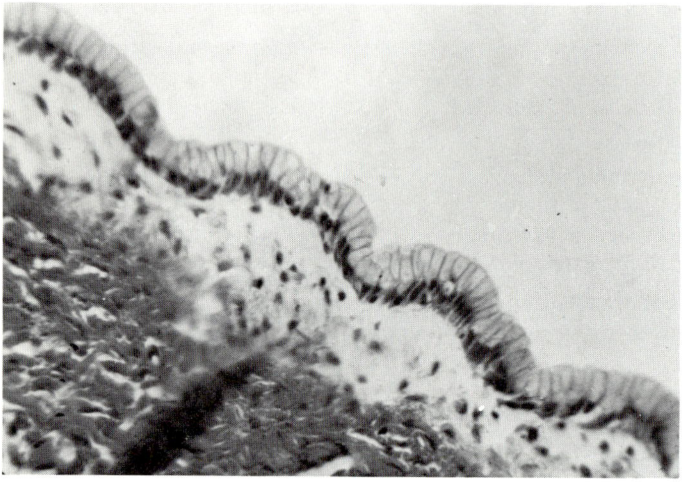

A

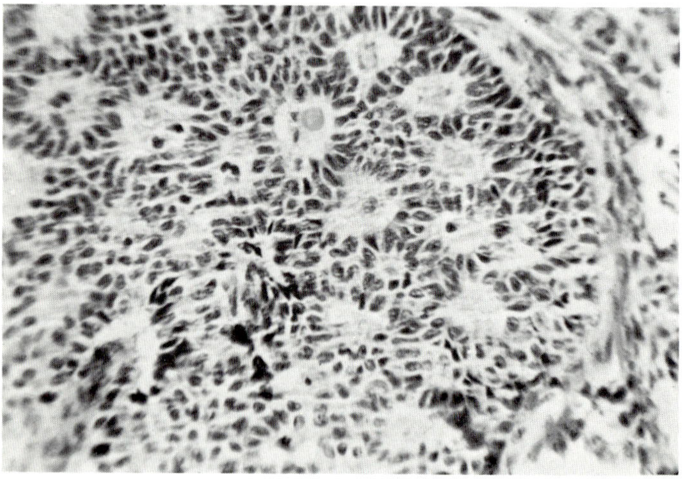

B

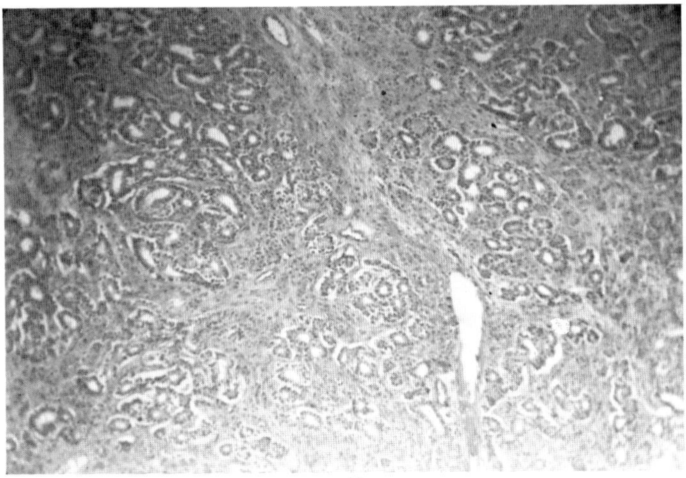

C

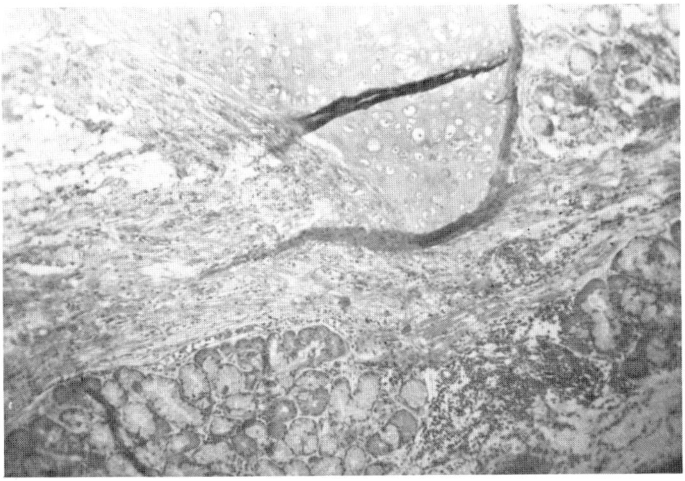

D

(A) Slide A
(B) Slide B
(C) Slide C
(D) Slide D
(E) None of the above

204. Granulosa cell tumor
205. Arrhenoblastoma
206. Benign cystic teratoma
207. Mucinous cystadenoma

Oncology

Answers

102. The answer is D. *(Novak, ed 7. pp 600-604. Rutledge, pp 139-142.)* The history, clinical picture, and tissue sample of the woman described are characteristic of hydatidiform mole. Initial symptoms usually include an enlarged-for-dates uterus and heavy vaginal bleeding. Hydatidiform mole is 10 times as common in the Far East as in North America. The tissue sample shows a villus with hydropic changes and no vessels. Grossly, these lesions appear as small, clear clusters of grapelike vesicles.

103. The answer is E. *(Rutledge, pp 262-264.)* Young women whose mothers ingested diethylstilbestrol during pregnancy are more apt to develop clear cell adenocarcinoma than other types of vaginal carcinoma. Although squamous carcinomas are the most common tumors of the vagina, they usually occur in women over the age of 40. Two rare vaginal carcinomas are papillary adenocarcinoma, which primarily affects older women, and carcinoma of the infantile vagina, which histologically resembles an endodermal sinus tumor of the ovary. Adenosquamous carcinomas usually are found in the uterus and less frequently in the cervix.

104. The answer is B. *(Novak, ed 7. pp 60-64.)* Carcinoma of the vagina, which occurs most frequently in women in their fifties and sixties, is most commonly epidermoid in origin and only rarely takes the form of adenocarcinoma. In addition, secondary carcinoma occurs much more frequently than primary carcinoma. The upper half of the anterior and posterior vaginal walls is most apt to be the site of vaginal carcinoma.

105. The answer is B. *(DiSaia, pp 114-116.)* The most important prognostic factor for Stage I endometrial carcinoma (carcinoma confined to the corpus uteri) is the grade, or degree of differentiation, of the tumor. Grade 1 tumors are well differentiated and are associated with a five-year survival rate of greater than 80 percent; Grade 3 tumors are poorly differentiated and are associated with a five-year survival rate of less than 45 percent. The depth of myometrial invasion and the involvement of pelvic lymph nodes correlate inversely with the degree of differentiation. Older women tend to have less well-differentiated tumors and therefore a poorer chance of survival.

106. The answer is D. *(Rutledge, pp 99-100, 110.)* Endometrial carcinoma involving the cervix is significant even if present only as microscopic disease. The lymphatic drainage of the uterine corpus is primarily by way of the lymphatics that follow the ovarian vessels. Because involvement of the cervix allows the cancer to metastasize via the parametrial lymphatics, five-year survival rate is reduced (regardless of the volume of tumor present) and intense radiotherapeutic treatment is required. Hysterectomy need not be excluded from the management program.

107. The answer is C. *(Rutledge, pp 106-107.)* Hysterectomy is the primary mode of treatment for women who have endometrial carcinoma confined to the uterine corpus. External beam and intracavitary radiation have been employed to help reduce central and pelvic recurrences of the cancer. Progestin therapy is used routinely as primary treatment of women who have advanced disease or recurrent carcinoma, and chemotherapy is used for patients whose tumors have failed to respond to other forms of therapy.

108. The answer is C. *(Brady, Gynecol Oncol 2[1974]: 314-323.)* Postmenopausal bleeding is the most common presenting symptom of women who have endometrial carcinoma. Because this warning signal is present even in the earliest stage of the disease, early diagnosis and treatment are possible. In fact, approximately 70 percent of affected women have Stage I disease when they first seek treatment.

109. The answer is D. *(MacMahon, Gynecol Oncol 2[1974]: 122-129.)* Pelvic irradiation, employed, for example, in the treatment of women who have cervical cancer, seems to be a contributory factor in the development of anaplastic endometrial carcinoma and mixed mesodermal carcinoma. Ingestion of conjugated estrogens or sequential birth-control pills has most often been associated with well-differentiated adenocarcinomas. Intrauterine devices and combined birth-control pills have not been associated with uterine malignancies.

110. The answer is E. *(Rutledge, pp 112-113.)* Cystic glandular hyperplasia progresses to endometrial carcinoma in only one to two percent of cases. Although some physicians consider it a precursor to adenocarcinoma, cystic hyperplasia is usually thought to antecede adenomatous hyperplasia, which then progresses to endometrial carcinoma in 5 to 15 percent of cases. For most patients, observation is the appropriate mode of management.

111. The answer is B. *(Rutledge, pp 124-128.)* Progestins have been employed successfully in the treatment of women who have recurrent endometrial carcinoma. In many series, response rates of 30 to 40 percent have been noted. The most frequently employed agents have been hydroxyprogesterone caproate (Delalutin) and medroxyprogesterone acetate (Provera). Single-agent chemotherapy with nonhormonal agents has produced disappointing responses in patients affected by advanced or recurrent endometrial carcinoma.

112. The answer is A. *(Rutledge, p 132.)* Leiomyosarcomas are the most common sarcomas of the uterus. They are discovered most frequently during a histologic examination of a leiomyomatous uterus and are often clinically and grossly indistinguishable from benign leiomyoma. A rapid enlargement of a leiomyomatous uterus may be the only indication of the presence of a sarcoma.

113. The answer is A. *(Novak, ed 7. p 203.)* Carcinoma of the ovary is the most common cause of metastatic adenocarcinoma of the uterus. Metastases from other, more distant sites, such as the stomach, also can give rise, though less often, to this lesion.

114. The answer is B. *(Novak, ed 7. pp 200-201.)* The belief that adenoacanthoma of the uterus is a combination of malignant tumors generally has been discarded. Current investigators feel that this tumor represents an adenocarcinoma with squamous metaplastic changes. When compared stage to stage, adenoacanthoma and adenocarcinoma have similar prognoses.

115. The answer is A. *(DiSaia, pp 147-148.)* Ovarian neoplasms arise more commonly from coelomic epithelium than from any other source. Many tumors of this group include epithelium that histologically resembles endocervical, endometrial, or fallopian-tube epithelium (giving rise respectively to mucinous, endometrioid, and serous carcinomas). Other, less common ovarian tumors of coelomic epithelial origin include mesonephroid carcinoma, Brenner tumors, mixed mesodermal tumors, and carcinosarcomas. Epithelial tumors frequently contain mixed cell types; categorization of these tumors is according to the cell type that predominates.

116. The answer is B. *(Novak, ed 7. pp 281-285.)* Mixed mesodermal tumors (mesenchymomas) of the uterus are similar to endometrial sarcoma. The combined incidence of these two types of malignancy is no higher than 0.5 percent. Although mixed mesodermal tumors occur most frequently in postmenopausal women, one variant, sarcoma botryoides, can develop in young children. Prognosis is poor, with a five-year survival rate of 26 to 28 percent being the highest reported. Maternal ingestion of estrogen during pregnancy has not, as yet, been associated with the development of mixed mesodermal tumors.

117. The answer is C. *(Novak, ed 7. p 431.)* The tissue specimen illustrated represents struma ovarii, which is composed of aberrant thyroid tissue that is frequently active and which is associated with mature cystic teratomas. The woman described manifests symptoms of thyrotoxicosis, such as diarrhea, rapid pulse, and weight loss; though not reported, her serum thyroxine levels would be elevated. The pathologic picture is characterized by thyroid tissue with large acini filled with colloid.

118. The answer is A. *(Rutledge, pp 159-160, 162.)* Ovarian carcinoma, though the third most common malignancy of gynecologic origin (after endometrial and cervical carcinoma), is associated with the highest mortality rate among the common gynecologic malignancies. The inability of routine screening tests to diagnose this malignancy in an early stage, in contrast to the efficacy of the Pap smear in detecting cervical cancer, is chiefly responsible for the high mortality rate. Most patients have advanced disease by the time their symptoms appear. Environmental, cultural, socioeconomic, and dietary factors all may play a role in the development of ovarian cancer.

119. The answer is C. *(Young, Sem Oncol 2[1975]:267-276.)* Alkylating agents, including melphalan, cyclophosphamide, chlorambucil, and triethylenethiophosphoramide, are useful in treating women who have ovarian epithelial tumors; objective response rates (partial and complete remissions) approach 50 percent in most series. Other agents that are currently being investigated and appear to be effective in the management of these women include doxorubicin (Adriamycin), hexamethylmelamine, and cis-platinum. Prospective randomized trials are underway to evaluate new single-agent treatments for women with ovarian cancer.

120. The answer is E. *(DiSaia, p 140.)* Approximately 70 percent of women who have ovarian cancer present with abdominal distension, and 50 percent present with abdominal pain. Gastrointestinal symptoms, which occur in about 20 percent of affected women, often are secondary to the development of ascites. Urinary-tract symptoms, due to the pressure exerted by a rapidly growing mass, and abnormal vaginal bleeding are the initial symptoms of ovarian cancer in 15 percent of affected women.

121. The answer is D. *(DiSaia, p 11.)* The International Federation of Gynecology and Obstetrics (FIGO) staging of primary ovarian carcinoma is in four categories: Stage I (with substages a to c), in which growth is limited to one or both ovaries and in which ascites can be present (Stage Ic); Stage II (with substages a, b, and c), in which carcinoma shows pelvic extension; Stage III, in which intraperitoneal metastasis is widespread; and Stage IV, in which the cancer has metastasized outside the peritoneal cavity. Disease that is thought to be, but not proven to be, ovarian carcinoma is defined as a special category. The FIGO staging is based on both clinical examination and surgical exploration.

122. The answer is C. *(DiSaia, pp 142-144.)* Benign cystic teratomas (dermoid cysts) of the ovary usually appear as anterior cul-de-sac masses that are mobile and unilateral. Serous carcinoma of the ovary, when diagnosed, usually is in an advanced stage and is a fixed, solid mass. Urachal cysts are midline structures and very infrequently diagnosed. Intraligamentous fibroids usually occur in older women, and diverticular abscesses are fixed masses associated with gastrointestinal symptoms.

123. The answer is E. *(Rutledge, pp 164-166.)* Peritoneal seeding is the major mode of spread of ovarian neoplasms. Ovarian malignancies also may extend locally to adjoining structures, such as the uterus, fallopian tubes, pelvic peritoneum, bladder peritoneum, and serosa of the sigmoid colon. Although dissemination by lymphatic and hematogenous routes does occur, it is of lesser importance than peritoneal seeding in producing symptoms and eventually causing death.

124. The answer is B. *(DiSaia, p 160.)* Mesonephric (clear cell) carcinoma of the ovary is thought to arise from paramesonephric coelomic epithelium and not from mesonephric embryonic rests. It represents approximately 5 percent of ovarian epithelial carcinomas, and affected women have a five-year survival of approximately 50 percent. Pelvic endometriosis occurs in at least one-fourth of women who have mesonephric carcinoma of the ovary. Endometrioid areas are seen not infrequently in association with mesonephric cancer.

125. The answer is E. *(Novak, ed 7. pp 394-404.)* Brenner tumors of the ovary generally are benign, slow-growing, and asymptomatic. Size varies widely; although many are microscopic, some may grow to be quite large (one tumor weighing more than 19 pounds has been reported). "Walthard rests," which are nests of epithelial cells surrounded by mesenchymal tissue, are diagnostic of Brenner tumor. Nuclei of the epithelial cells are grooved longitudinally and, as a result, are referred to as "coffee-bean" nuclei.

126. The answer is A. *(DiSaia, pp 164-165.)* Radioisotopes are beta-particle emitters whose depth of effective radiation is limited to a few millimeters. Because of their limited range, they are not employed routinely in management of women who have advanced ovarian malignancies. However, it has been shown that survivability may be significantly enhanced if radioisotopes are used in women in whom a malignant ovarian cyst has ruptured intraperitoneally, provided there is no other evidence of intraperitoneal malignancy.

127. The answer is E. *(DiSaia, p 164.)* The survivability of women who have ovarian carcinoma varies inversely with the amount of residual tumor left after the initial surgery. At the time of laparotomy, a maximum effort should be made to determine the sites of tumor spread and excise all resectable tumor. Although the uterus and ovary may appear grossly normal, there is a relatively high incidence of occult metastases to these organs; for this reason, they should be removed during the initial surgery.

128. The answer is C. *(Rutledge, pp 188-189.)* Postoperative whole-abdomen irradiation combined with additional radiation to the pelvis has produced the highest five-year survival rates of any treatment used for patients who have Stage II epithelial ovarian tumors. Because ovarian tumor cells tend to exfoliate and spread throughout the abdominal cavity, irradiation of the pelvis alone is insufficient treatment. The liver and kidneys must be shielded during at least part of the external beam therapy, and bowel injury may be a late sequela.

129. The answer is B. *(Herbst, Clin Obstet Gynecol 18[1975]:185-194.)* Irregular vaginal bleeding has been the most frequent presenting symptom of women who have clear cell adenocarcinoma of the vagina. Routine screening of women who were exposed in utero to diethylstilbestrol can detect a significant number of cases of asymptomatic adenocarcinoma. Asymptomatic patients tend to have smaller lesions and better prognoses.

130. The answer is D. *(Young, Sem Oncol 2[1975]:267-276.)* Intraperitoneal administration of alkylating agents is not as effective as systemic administration in treating women who have ovarian cancer. No evidence now exists that any particular alkylating agent or dose schedule is superior to any other. Tests comparing the effectiveness of high-dose intravenous cyclophosphamide to standard doses of orally administered melphalan showed no difference in response but a significant increase in toxicity. Patients who previously had been treated with radiation therapy had poorer response rates than patients who received chemotherapy as primary treatment.

131. The answer is C. *(Herbst, Clin Obstet Gynecol 18[1975]: 185-194.)* A hooded cervix, a "cockscomb" cervix, and cervical pseudopolyps are common structural changes associated with in utero exposure to diethylstilbestrol or chemically related nonsteroidal estrogens. Cervical erosions are almost always found in affected individuals, and vaginal adenosis is frequently present. Carcinomas of the vagina are much less frequently diagnosed.

132. The answer is A. *(Novak, ed 7. p 133.)* The majority of deaths from cervical cancer result from the effects of local extension. These effects include urinary insufficiency, intestinal obstruction, and debility and malnutrition. Approximately two-fifths of all women who die of cervical cancer have evidence of extrapelvic metastasis; spread of the tumor, presumably via the bloodstream, occasionally involves distant organs, including the liver, spine, and brain.

133. The answer is C. *(Novak, ed 7. pp 106, 109.)* Carcinoma in situ of the cervix involves the entire squamous epithelium, which is displaced by cells that are similar to those of invasive carcinoma. Stratification is completely lost, but no evidence of stromal or lymphatic invasion has been noted. Although carcinoma in situ is generally considered to precede development of frank invasive cancer, the lesion has been reported to regress and disappear on occasion.

134. The answer is D. *(Novak, ed 7. p 117.)* The FIGO classification is the most widely accepted staging for cervical carcinoma. Stage 0 is pre-invasive and represents carcinoma in situ. Stage I disease is confined to the cervix; in Stage Ia, diagnosis of the malignancy cannot be revealed by clinical examination (Stage Ib encompasses all other cases). Although Stage II carcinoma extends beyond the cervix, it does not involve the pelvic wall or the lower one-third of the vagina. Obvious parametrial involvement may be absent (Stage IIa) or present (Stage IIb). Stage III carcinoma extends to the pelvic wall and the lower one-third of the vagina. Stage IV disease extends beyond the true pelvis.

135. The answer is B. *(Novak, ed 7. p 130.)* Because the squamous epithelia of the vaginal portio and the cervix are directly contiguous, the portio is more likely to show secondary involvement with cervical cancer than any other site. Extension to the corpus uteri and parametrium can occur in more advanced stages of the disease. However, it is lymphatic spread, rather than local extension, that makes control and treatment of cervical cancer so difficult.

136. The answer is C. *(Gunning, Obstet Gynecol Survey 31[1976]: 827-833.)* Clear cell adenocarcinoma of the cervix has been reported to occur, although somewhat less frequently than clear cell carcinoma of the vagina, in women exposed to diethylstilbestrol in utero. Adenosis of the vagina has been associated with nearly one-third of clear cell carcinomas of the cervix but with 90 percent of clear cell carcinomas of the vagina. Microglandular hyperplasia is a benign lesion whose development is linked to the use of oral contraceptives.

137. The answer is A. *(Hilgers, Gynecol Oncol 2[1974]: 460-475.)* Gestational trophoblastic disease is the neoplasm most sensitive to appropriate chemotherapeutic agents, such as methotrexate and actinomycin D. Treatment of women who have nonmetastatic gestational trophoblastic disease is almost 100 percent successful and allows reproductive function to be preserved. Cure rates for metastatic disease approach 90 percent.

138. The answer is A. *(Hilgers, Gynecol Oncol 2[1974]: 460-475.)* The condition of women who have hydatidiform moles but no evidence of metastatic disease should be followed routinely by human chorionic gonadotropin (HCG) titers. Most authorities agree that prophylactic chemotherapy should not be employed in the routine management of women having hydatidiform moles, because 85 to 90 percent of affected patients will require no further treatment. For a young woman in whom preservation of reproductive function is important, surgery is not routinely indicated.

139. The answer is E. *(Rutledge, p 143.)* Adnexal masses are present in approximately one-third of women who have hydatidiform moles. These masses represent theca-lutein cysts that result from human chorionic gonadotropin stimulation. The cysts tend to be bilateral and usually require no therapeutic intervention, unless they undergo torsion, an unusual event.

140. The answer is B. *(Hilgers, Gynecol Oncol 2[1974]:460-475.)* Ultrasonography is the most reliable method for early diagnosis of hydatidiform mole. Amniography, another useful method, requires percutaneous insertion of a needle into the uterine cavity and injection of a radiopaque contrast dye. A plain film of the abdomen cannot demonstrate a hydatidiform mole, and elevated HCG titers would be nondiagnostic. Pelvic arteriography would expose an accompanying normal fetus to high doses of radiation.

141. The answer is E. *(Hilgers, Gynecol Oncol 2[1974]: 460-475.)* Viable trophoblastic tissue produces human chorionic gonadotropin (HCG). The presence of elevated HCG titers confirms the presence of trophoblastic tissue and allows careful monitoring of the effectiveness of chemotherapy. Theca-lutein cysts tend to decrease in size following evacuation of a hydatidiform mole despite the persistence of viable trophoblastic cells; and normal cyclic menstruation may reappear in spite of continued disease activity. Chest x-ray changes often persist for several months after HCG titers have returned to normal.

142. The answer is D. *(Rutledge, p 216.)* Approximately one-fourth of women affected by extramammary Paget's disease of the vulva have apocrine gland carcinoma. The finding of an apocrine gland carcinoma usually is considered an indication for regional lymphadenectomy. Metastatic disease in regional lymph nodes is associated with an extremely poor prognosis.

143. The answer is D. *(Novak, ed 7. pp 37-40.)* The woman described in the question has invasive squamous cell carcinoma of the vulva, with penetration below the basement membrane. The squamous epithelial cells have an irregular shape and an abnormal nuclear-cytoplasmic ratio and show an increased number of mitotic figures. Tuberculosis of the vulva is characterized by multinucleated giant cells; Bowen's disease tissue does not show invasion below the basement membrane; and Paget's disease of the vulva, which is rare, is characterized by Paget cells, large cells that have abundant granular cytoplasm and basophilic nuclei.

144. The answer is E. *(DiSaia, pp 224-226.)* Patients who have invasive vulvar carcinoma usually are treated surgically. If the lesions are unilateral, are not associated with fixed or ulcerated inguinal lymph nodes, and do not involve the urethra, vagina, anus, or rectum, then treatment usually consists of radical vulvectomy and bilateral inguinal lymphadenectomy. If inguinal lymph nodes show evidence of metastatic disease, bilateral pelvic lymphadenectomy is usually performed. Radiation therapy, though not a routine part of the management of women who have early vulvar carcinoma, is employed (as an alternative to pelvic exenteration with radical vulvectomy) in the treatment of women who have local advanced carcinoma.

145. The answer is A (1, 2, 3). *(Novak, ed 7. pp 204-211.)* Adenocarcinoma of the uterus has been found to be associated with such gynecologic factors as late menopause, anovulation, and a poor fertility index. Prolonged estrogen therapy, too, has been implicated in the development of uterine cancer. Adenomatous hyperplasia of the endometrium is not only associated with adenocarcinoma but also widely considered to be a precancerous lesion.

146. The answer is B (1, 3). *(Rutledge, p 101.)* Recent evidence suggests that adenosquamous carcinoma of the endometrium has a poorer prognosis than either adenocarcinoma or adenoacanthoma of the endometrium. It has yet to be resolved whether the poorer prognosis associated with adenosquamous lesions is due to the population of malignant squamous cells or to the poorly differentiated adenomatous elements, which normally carry a poor prognosis. Adenoacanthoma, which is characterized by benign metaplasia of squamous epithelium, has a prognosis similar to that of other adenocarcinomas of the endometrium. Adenosquamous tumors tend to occur more frequently in older women.

147. The answer is E (all). *(Novak, ed 7. p 190.)* Although the carcinogenesis of endometrial cancer is still in dispute, several facts regarding its incidence are clear. The disease primarily affects women who have passed the menopause; on the average, endometrial cancer appears ten years later than the onset of cervical carcinoma. The fact that the frequency of this condition has been increasing certainly is due in part to the increased life span of American women. Most studies have revealed a five-year survival rate of about 75 percent for women who have endometrial cancer.

148. The answer is E (all). *(Novak, ed 7. pp 218-219.)* Successful treatment of endometrial carcinoma involves both radiation and surgery. Survival rates are related to the extent of the disease as follows: greater than 90 percent when the disease is limited to the endometrium; greater than 80 percent in the presence of superficial myometrial invasion; approximately 50 percent if there is extensive myometrial or cervical involvement; and 25 percent or less if extrauterine spread has occurred.

149. The answer is C (2, 4). *(Brady, Gynecol Oncol 2[1974]: 314-323.)* Intracavitary radium has been successfully employed as the primary mode of therapy for women who have surgically inoperable endometrial cancer and have small uteri with a well-differentiated tumor. Vaginal apical recurrences occur in 10 to 15 percent of affected women who were treated by hysterectomy alone; this incidence can be reduced significantly with the use of intravaginal radium. Because the effectiveness of intracavitary radium rapidly decreases as tissue depth increases, it is not a satisfactory treatment for women who have ovarian or pelvic sidewall metastases.

150. The answer is E (all). *(Brady, Gynecol Oncol 2[1974]: 314-323.)* The presence of factors associated with extrauterine spread of uterine malignancies is an ominous prognostic sign. These factors include an enlarged uterus, deep myometrial invasion, anaplastic adenocarcinoma, and gross extension to the cervix or fornices. Except for invasion of the myometrium, these factors usually can be determined before treatment is instituted and are indications for preoperative external beam radiation therapy; the presence of deep myometrial invasion, of course, can only be assessed in a hysterectomy specimen.

151. The answer is C (2, 4). *(MacMahon, Gynecol Oncol 2[1974]: 122-129.)* Carcinoma of the endometrium is unusual in women under the age of 40. It has been associated with Stein-Leventhal (polycystic ovary) syndrome and has been reported in patients who have had gonadal dysgenesis and who were treated with exogenous estrogen (diethylstilbestrol) for more than five years. Ovarian choriocarcinomas and dysgerminomas are not associated with a higher incidence of endometrial carcinoma.

152. The answer is E (all). *(MacMahon, Gynecol Oncol 2[1974]: 122-129.)* Endometrial carcinoma tends to occur in obese, diabetic women who undergo late-onset menopause and are nulliparous or have low parity. Other factors that may predispose to endometrial carcinoma include hypertension, cancer at other sites (e.g., ovary and breast), and familial history of this malignancy.

153. The answer is E (all). *(Rutledge, pp 108-109.)* Endometrial hyperplasia tends to develop in those women who also are at significant risk for developing adenocarcinoma of the endometrium. Hyperplasia is associated with unopposed estrogen stimulation of the endometrium, which occurs most often as a woman approaches menopause. However, it also may be associated with prolonged anovulation (as seen occasionally in postpartum women), with Stein-Leventhal syndrome, and with functioning ovarian tumors, such as granulosa-theca-cell tumor.

154. The answer is E (all). *(Rutledge, p 124.)* Patients who have well-differentiated tumors of the uterus generally have a better response to progestin than those women who have anaplastic tumors. Younger women tend to respond better than older women, due at least in part to the tendency of younger women to have well-differentiated tumors and older women to have more anaplastic tumors. Metastases to the lung respond more favorably to progestin therapy than large, fixed pelvic tumors.

155. The answer is B (1, 3). *(Novak, ed 7. p 198.)* Histologic grading is valuable both in describing adenocarcinoma of the uterus and in determining the prognosis. The Broders classification (grades I to IV) is the one most widely used; 75 to 100 percent of the cells in Grade I tumors are differentiated, while in Grade IV tumors (the most malignant) 75 to 100 percent of the cells are undifferentiated. The FIGO Cancer Committee has identified three grades of tumor: 1) highly differentiated; 2) differentiated with partly solid areas; and 3) predominantly solid or undifferentiated (the most malignant). Although myometrial invasion is very important in the prognosis of adenocarcinoma of the uterus, it is not a factor in the grading.

156. The answer is C (2, 4). *(Novak, ed 7. pp 203-204.)* Although the most common route of dissemination of adenocarcinoma of the body of the uterus is the lymphatics, this tumor spreads much less often than cervical malignancies and only rarely affects distant organs. Nearby surface structures are affected more frequently, and the cervix, bladder, and rectum can become involved in advanced cases. Direct extension, though not as common as lymphatic dissemination, also is important.

157. The answer is C (2, 4). *(DiSaia, p 141.)* Unilateral, cystic, mobile, and small (less than 10 cm) adnexal masses tend to be benign neoplasms. Masses that are bilateral, solid, fixed, and large, on the other hand, more characteristically are malignant and require prompt diagnostic evaluation and treatment. Ascites also is frequently associated with ovarian malignancies.

158. The answer is A (1, 2, 3). *(DiSaia, pp 142-145.)* A chest x-ray, an intravenous pyelogram, and a barium enema all are important in the evaluation of a woman suspected of having an ovarian malignancy. Chest x-rays can reveal occult metastases as well as pleural effusions, which frequently occur in advanced ovarian cancer. Pyelography can assess renal function and reveal ureteral obstruction or deviation as well as duplication of urinary-tract structures. Barium enemas can help distinguish a neoplastic or inflammatory process arising from the colon from extrinsic compression due to an ovarian tumor. A liver scan is not routinely performed, because ovarian cancer usually does not spread hematogenously; a scan is indicated only if liver function tests are abnormal or the liver is palpably enlarged.

159. The answer is E (all). *(DiSaia, p 146.)* Unsuspected ovarian tumors in women in the reproductive years may be discovered fortuitously during a laparotomy. Hemorrhagic ascites, surface excrescences on the ovary, peritoneal implants, intracystic papillations, bilateralism, adhesion to adjacent regions, and areas of hemorrhage and necrosis within the tumor all suggest that an ovarian tumor is malignant.

160. The answer is E (all). *(DiSaia, pp 146, 169.)* Conservation of reproductive potential or function should be a major consideration in the surgical management of children and of women in the reproductive years. An adequate intraoperative evaluation should include biopsy of the omentum, a biopsy of the uninvolved ovary, and peritoneal cytology; in addition, careful intra-abdominal exploration and biopsy of any abnormalities also should be performed. Although it is unnecessary to biopsy a grossly normal liver, the diaphragm must be examined closely, and any implants on the diaphragm should be biopsied.

161. The answer is E (all). *(Novak, ed 7. pp 367-387.)* Stromo-epithelial neoplasms, which comprise 75 to 80 percent of all primary ovarian cancers, may be of the following histologic types: serous, mucinous, endometrioid, and mesonephroid. These types may be thought of as forms of differentiated mesotheliomas. Serous lesions are the most common variety of ovarian cystomas, and mucinous tumors may become large enough to fill the abdomen. The prognosis for women who have endometrioid lesions, which metastasize only infrequently and are not considered to be very malignant, is good. Pure mesonephroid tumors are rare.

162. The answer is C (2, 4). *(DiSaia, pp 153-157.)* Epithelial ovarian tumors of low potential malignancy represent 15 percent of all epithelial ovarian tumors. Although they do not infiltrate destructively into the ovarian stroma, these borderline malignancies have been associated with late recurrences and death and may metastasize throughout the peritoneal cavity. Histologically, these tumors demonstrate proliferative activity, abnormal mitoses, and nuclear abnormalities. Ten-year survival rates of women who have Stage I tumors of low potential malignancy have been reported to be 95 percent.

163. The answer is A (1, 2, 3). *(DiSaia, pp 157-160.)* Serous carcinoma is the most common epithelial tumor of the ovary. Psammoma bodies can be seen in approximately 30 percent of these tumors; and bilateral involvement characterizes about one-third of all serous carcinomas. Although mesonephroid carcinomas tend to be associated with pelvic endometriosis, a similar association has not been demonstrated for serous carcinomas.

164. The answer is E (all). *(Rutledge, pp 167-169.)* Mucinous carcinomas of the ovary usually are diagnosed at an earlier stage than serous carcinomas and tend to be histologically well differentiated. This combination of diagnosis at an early stage (when the tumors frequently are unilateral) and well-differentiated histologic appearance is probably the reason that patients who have mucinous carcinoma have a better five-year survival rate than patients affected by serous carcinoma. Mucinous tumors of the ovary, which are less common than serous lesions, usually are lobulated and may grow to enormous proportions.

165. The answer is D (4). *(DiSaia, p 158.)* Endometrioid carcinoma of the ovary, which may be histologically indistinguishable from endometrial carcinoma, can undergo squamous metaplasia. Although it is associated with endometrial carcinoma in up to 30 percent of affected women, endometrioid carcinoma is felt to represent a primary, rather than a metastatic, lesion. Ovarian endometriosis may be present, but malignant transformation is not routinely demonstrated. The five-year survival rate approaches 50 percent for women who have endometrioid carcinoma of the ovary, a much higher rate than that associated with serous carcinoma.

166. The answer is E (all). *(DiSaia, pp 161-164.)* The extent (or stage) and the volume of a tumor are probably the most important prognostic considerations in the management of women who have ovarian epithelial carcinoma. However, on a stage-for-stage basis, women who have well-differentiated tumors have better prognoses than women who have poorly differentiated tumors. The presence of ascites or peritoneal washings that are cytologically positive for malignant cells decreases the five-year survival of affected women.

167. The answer is A (1, 2, 3). *(Rutledge, pp 178-179.)* If either the serosa of the liver or the peritoneum overlying the kidney is the site of metastatic ovarian carcinoma, external-beam radiation therapy is contraindicated, because these organs are extremely sensitive to radiation. In addition, the radiation doses necessary to control tumors of more than 2 cm in diameter are prohibitively high relative to the bowel. Other factors militating against the use of external-beam radiation therapy include metastasis to distant sites, clinically apparent ascites, but not pelvic retroperitoneal metastases.

168. The answer is A (1, 2, 3). *(Rutledge, pp 194-197.)* The histologic type of epithelial ovarian cancer does not appear to play a significant role in the progression or regression of disease between initial and "second look" surgery. Factors that are of prognostic significance include the volume of residual tumor left at the initial surgery, the number of courses of chemotherapy, and the presence of palpable tumor. The histologic grade of the initial tumor also is prognostically significant, because women who have well-differentiated tumors appear to respond better to chemotherapy than women affected by poorly differentiated tumors.

169. The answer is A (1, 2, 3). *(Novak, ed 7. p 367.)* Ovarian carcinoma is difficult to diagnose; cytologic smears of the vagina and cervix are of little value in identifying an ovarian malignancy. Approximately 12 to 20 percent of all primary genital-canal malignancies occur in the ovary, which is the third most common site of genital cancer. Although cervical cancer is more common, more deaths occur annually from ovarian cancer. More than 10,000 women die annually of ovarian cancer, which is the cause of death of at least 1 percent of all women older than 40 years. The cystic form of carcinoma of the ovary is about twice as common as the solid variety.

170. The answer is B (1, 3). *(Herbst, Clin Obstet Gynecol 18[1975]: 185-194.)* A maternal history of ingestion of nonsteroidal synthetic estrogens, including hexestrol, dienestrol, and diethylstilbestrol, has been associated with 65 percent of the women who have developed clear cell adenocarcinoma of the vagina. Development of the neoplasm has not been linked with intrauterine exposure to progestins (such as ethinylestrenol and medroxyprogesterone acetate). Although the amount of drug ingested does not seem to be a significant factor, all patients found to have clear cell adenocarcinoma were exposed prior to the eighteenth week of gestation.

171. The answer is A (1, 2, 3). *(Rutledge, pp 259-260.)* Squamous carcinoma of the vagina, which tends to occur in older women and is most frequently located on the posterior wall of the vagina, is the most common type of vaginal carcinoma. Carcinoma in the lower one-third of the vagina can metastasize by way of vulvar lymphatics; tumors situated in the upper vagina may spread via cervical lymphatics. Carcinoma in situ of the vagina is often multifocal.

172. The answer is E (all). *(Novak, ed 7. p 63.)* A number of young women whose mothers were treated with diethylstilbestrol during pregnancy (particularly before the eighteenth week of gestation) have been found to have adenocarcinoma of the vagina. The tumors of these women, who generally are in their late teens or early twenties, usually are located in the middle third or outer third of the vagina. Microscopic examination reveals that the malignancies are clear cell tumors with papillary projections; when viewed by electron microscopy, these tumors show evidence of a müllerian origin.

173. The answer is A (1, 2, 3). *(Novak, ed 7. p 110.)* Carcinoma of the cervix is considered to be invasive when the basement membrane has been pierced, allowing cancer cells into the stroma. Histologic evidence of abnormal cell maturation and presence of cancer cells in the lymphatics also indicate invasive disease. Involvement of endocervical glands is not indicative of invasion.

174. The answer is C (2, 4). *(Novak, ed 7. p 114.)* Diagnosis of microinvasion of the cervix is made if the disease process is limited to the 5 mm beneath the basal layer. Invasion of the stroma, whether or not the lymphatics also are involved, is the cause of death of 1 to 2 percent of women who die of cervical carcinoma. Extensive surgery or radiation is required once stromal or lymphatic invasion is identified.

175. The answer is B (1, 3). *(Novak, ed 7. pp 34-37. Romney, pp 932, 966.)* The lesion illustrated is Paget's disease. Paget cells are large, vacuolated cells with a distinct, basophilic nucleus. Paget's disease is a carcinoma of apocrine sweat glands, which are found in the vulva and the areola of the breast. Treatment for women who have vulvar Paget's disease is vulvectomy.

176. The answer is D (4). *(Novak, ed 7. pp 125-130.)* Adenocarcinoma of the cervix, which occurs less commonly than the epidermoid type, accounts for approximately 4 to 5 percent of all cervical carcinomas. Adenocarcinoma usually occurs in younger women, and epidermoid in older. Although adenocarcinoma characteristically arises within the cervical canal and epidermoid cancer usually arises in the region of the external os, both types of malignancy can occur in either location. Clear cell (mesonephroid) carcinoma, which can arise from mesonephric remnants, is a rare type of adenocarcinoma.

177. The answer is C (2, 4). *(Hilgers, Gynecol Oncol 2[1974]:460-475.)* The first successful treatment regimen for women who had gestational trophoblastic disease consisted of single-agent methotrexate chemotherapy. Subsequent studies combining methotrexate, actinomycin D, and an alkylating agent were successful in treating methotrexate-resistant trophoblastic disease. Actinomycin D, then studied as a single agent, proved to be as effective as methotrexate; in addition, it was not hampered by cross-resistance in methotrexate-resistant tumors and was safer to use in women who had impaired liver function.

178. The answer is B (1, 3). *(Hilgers, Gynecol Oncol 2[1974]:460-475.)* Women whose trophoblastic disease has metastasized to the brain or liver have poorer prognoses and require more intense treatment than women who have lung or vaginal metastases. The selection of chemotherapeutic regimens is based on this and other prognostic factors; localized radiation therapy frequently is employed to reduce the risk of hemorrhage when brain and liver metastases are present.

179. The answer is A (1, 2, 3). *(Hilgers, Gynecol Oncol 2[1974]: 460-475.)* The term "gestational trophoblastic disease" refers to a group of neoplasms, such as hydatidiform mole, choriocarcinoma, and chorioadenoma destruens, that arise as the result of pregnancy. Although the pregnancy itself can be affected (e.g., hydatidiform mole), neoplasms of this group also can be diagnosed following normal intrauterine pregnancies, ectopic pregnancies, or abortions. Chorioadenoma destruens is a molar lesion that has invaded the myometrium; choriocarcinoma, which can occur anywhere in the uterus, is composed of malignant trophoblastic cells that metastasize easily. The term "gestational trophoblastic disease" distinguishes such neoplasms from primary trophoblastic neoplasms arising in the ovary or testes.

180. The answer is D (4). *(Hilgers, Gynecol Oncol 2[1974]: 460-475.)* The classification of gestational trophoblastic disease is based both on its histologic appearance (including villus-structure retention) as well as on the location of its metastases. This method of classification has not been found to be a reliable indicator of prognosis or management and does not provide a means of estimating the likelihood of complete remission. A better classification distinguishes between metastatic and nonmetastatic gestational trophoblastic disease as well as between gestational and nongestational trophoblastic disease, such as primary choriocarcinoma of the ovary.

181. The answer is B (1, 3). *(Hilgers, Gynecol Oncol 2[1974]: 460-475.)* Choriocarcinoma, which is made up of anaplastic and hyperplastic cytotrophoblastic and syncytial constituents, usually metastasizes by hematogenous routes and can produce symptoms due to metastasis to nonreproductive organs several years following the last known pregnancy. The most common site of distant metastasis is the lung. Approximately half of choriocarcinomas are preceded by hydatidiform mole; the other 50 percent may have been preceded by abortions, ectopic pregnancies, or even term pregnancies.

182. The answer is A (1, 2, 3). *(Hilgers, Gynecol Oncol 2[1974]: 460-475.)* Women who have had gestational trophoblastic disease for less than four months, whose 24-hour urine titers of human chorionic gonadotropin (HCG) are less than 100,000 international units, and whose metastases are limited to the vagina or lungs have a 95 percent cure rate and are thus considered low-risk patients. Patients whose disease has lasted for more than four months, whose HCG titer is greater than 100,000 international units per 24 hours, and who have liver or brain metastases, on the other hand, are classified as high-risk.

183. The answer is B (1, 3). *(Hilgers, Gynecol Oncol 2[1974]: 460-475.)* Single-agent chemotherapy usually is instituted if levels of HCG have remained elevated eight weeks after evacuation of a hydatidiform mole. Approximately half of the patients who have persistently high HCG titers will develop malignant sequelae. If HCG titers rise following molar evacuation, single-agent chemotherapy should be instituted, provided that the trophoblastic disease has not metastasized to the liver or brain. The presence of such metastases usually requires initiation of combination chemotherapy.

184. The answer is B (1, 3). *(Rutledge, pp 213-217.)* Squamous carcinoma is the most common malignancy of the vulva and accounts for approximately 85 percent of all cases of the disease. It is a disease of older women (three-fourths of affected patients are at least 50 years of age at the time of diagnosis). Carcinomas of Bartholin's glands comprise only about 1 percent of carcinomas of the vulva. Current information suggests that vulvar dystrophies, including leukoplakia, infrequently precede development of invasive vulvar carcinoma.

185. The answer is C (2, 4). *(Novak, ed 7. pp 37-38.)* Although primary carcinoma of the vulva is considered a disease of the elderly, the average age of affected women falls to about 40 years if its development is preceded by granulomatous disease. The initial appearance of this lesion often is inconspicuous. Microscopic examination commonly reveals large, highly differentiated spinal cells that typically form "pearls" and invade the stroma. Most of the tumor's extension is local; widespread metastasis to distant regions is infrequent. Of all genital cancers, carcinoma of the vulva ranks only behind uterine and ovarian cancer in incidence. Vulvar cancer represents three to four percent of all malignant genital lesions.

186. The answer is A (1, 2, 3). *(Rutledge, pp 217, 222.)* Regional lymph-node metastases are present in approximately 38 percent of patients whose vulvar lesions are greater than 2 cm in diameter but only 15 percent of patients whose lesions are less than 2 cm in diameter. Involvement of the anus or vagina is associated with an increased likelihood of regional node disease. Also, involvement of midline structures may result in bilateral regional lymph-node metastasis. Extension to the perineum without involvement of the anus or vagina does not increase the incidence of regional lymph-node metastasis.

187. The answer is B (1, 3). *(DiSaia, pp 227-228.)* Epidermoid carcinoma, the most common variety of vulvar cancer, usually is diagnosed at a less advanced stage than adenocarcinoma, which is a rare tumor that most often arises from Bartholin's glands. Epidermoid carcinoma tends to affect women who, on the average, are older than those affected by adenocarcinoma. Patients who have epidermoid carcinoma of the vulva have been noted to have an increased incidence of epidermoid carcinoma of the cervix.

188. The answer is B (1, 3). *(Novak, ed 7. pp 314-317.)* Because affected women have a low five-year survival rate, primary tubal carcinoma is thought to be highly malignant; this relationship, however, may be due more to delayed discovery of the tumor than to its malignant potential. Primary tubal carcinoma accounts for only about 0.2 to 0.5 percent of primary malignancies of the genital tract. Microscopically, these tumors present a papillary or papillary-alveolar pattern. Bilateral involvement occurs in about one-fourth of affected patients.

189. The answer is A (1, 2, 3). *(DiSaia, pp 254-256.)* Vaginal discharge, abdominal pain, and the presence of an adnexal mass comprise the clinical triad of signs and symptoms seen in approximately two-thirds of patients who have carcinoma of the fallopian tube. The diagnosis of fallopian tube carcinoma, the rarest of the carcinomas of the female genital tract, is rarely made preoperatively. This carcinoma also should be suspected in postmenopausal women who are thought to have pelvic inflammatory disease or who have vaginal bleeding for which no obvious cause is demonstrable by endometrial curettage.

190. The answer is B (1, 3). *(Novak, ed 7. pp 406-407.)* Hydrothorax and ascites are the characteristic features of Meigs' syndrome. It is believed that fluid accumulates in the thorax by permeating through diaphragmatic lymphatics. First described in association with ovarian fibromas, Meigs' syndrome also can be seen in combination with Brenner tumors, thecomas, granulosa cell tumors, and other solid ovarian tumors; large subserous myomas, however, are not associated with development of this syndrome.

191. The answer is E (all). *(DiSaia, p 189.)* Most ovarian neoplasms in children are of germ cell origin, and about half of these tumors are malignant. Functioning ovarian tumors have been reported to produce precocious puberty in about 2 percent of affected patients. Epithelial tumors of the ovary, which are quite rare in prepubertal girls, are benign in approximately 90 percent of all cases.

192. The answer is C (2, 4). *(DiSaia, pp 188-189.)* Ovarian neoplasms associated with pregnancy are usually benign; only 3 to 6 percent are found to be malignant. The neoplasms are most often unilateral when malignant. It has been estimated that 10 percent of ovarian masses discovered during pregnancy represent an enlarged, cystic corpus luteum. Transplacental spread of ovarian carcinoma to the fetus has not been documented.

193. The answer is B (1, 3). *(DiSaia, pp 212-213.)* Sarcoma botryoides is characterized grossly by a polypoid mass that fills the vagina and frequently protrudes through the vaginal introitus. The usual presenting symptom is vaginal discharge or bleeding. Sarcoma botryoides, which occurs most frequently in children, is usually multicentric in origin. Cartilagenous and osseous elements are not commonly found, although rhabdomyoblastic elements are.

194-198. The answers are: 194-B, 195-A, 196-D, 197-D, 198-A. *(DiSaia, pp 172-173, 175-177. Rutledge, pp 202-204. Smith, Cancer 36[1975]: 669-674.)* Of the approximately 1 percent of dermoid cysts that undergo malignant degeneration, 80 percent become squamous carcinoma. Other forms of malignant degeneration of dermoid cysts include adenocarcinoma, sarcoma, melanoma, and thyroid carcinoma associated with struma ovarii. Most cases of malignant degeneration of dermoid cysts appear after the menopause.

Because dysgerminomas are extremely radiosensitive, radiotherapy alone is used in the management of patients who have metastatic dysgerminoma. There is a strong tendency for dysgerminomas to spread through the lymphatic system, and lymphangiograms may be very useful in defining patterns of spread and radiotherapy fields. Conservative treatment (unilateral salpingo-oophorectomy) is justified only for patients who have small tumors (less than 10 cm) that are unilateral and intact, who have no evidence of metastatic tumor, and in whom preservation of fertility is important. Dysgerminomas frequently arise in gonadoblastomas (about half of all reported cases of gonadoblastomas are associated with dysgerminomas). Choriocarcinoma and embryonal carcinoma are less frequently associated with gonadoblastoma, a benign lesion of individuals who usually have some degree of gonadal dysgenesis.

Embryonal carcinoma is an extremely malignant ovarian neoplasm. Women who have embryonal carcinoma of the ovary frequently have elevated serum alpha-fetoprotein levels. If present, this protein may be used as a tumor-specific index in following the progress of the disease and assessing therapy. Regardless of the stage of the disease, affected women are treated routinely with combination chemotherapy: vincristine, actinomycin D, and cyclophosphamide. Patients treated with radiation therapy or single-agent chemotherapy rarely survive for prolonged periods of time. Combination chemotherapy, on the other hand, has produced long-term remissions; and in one small series of patients, no residual tumor was reported at second-look surgery.

199-203. The answers are: 199-B, 200-A, 201-A, 202-D, 203-C. *(DiSaia, pp 176-177, 181-185. Rutledge, pp 206-207.)* Sertoli-Leydig cell tumors, which represent less than 1 percent of ovarian tumors, may produce symptoms of virilization. Histologically, they resemble fetal testes; clinically, they must be distinguished from other functioning ovarian neoplasms as well as from tumors of the adrenal glands. Recurrences of Sertoli-Leydig cell tumors, which seem to have a low malignant potential, usually appear within three years of the original diagnosis.

Granulosa and theca cell tumors often are associated with excessive estrogen production, which may cause pseudoprecocious puberty, postmenopausal bleeding, or menorrhagia. These tumors are associated with endometrial carcinoma in 15 percent of patients. Because these tumors are quite friable, affected women frequently present with symptoms caused by tumor rupture and intraperitoneal bleeding. Granulosa tumors are low-grade malignancies that tend to recur more than five years after the initial diagnosis. Because their malignant potential is impossible to predict histologically, long-term follow-up is mandatory for these patients. Recurrences have been reported as late as 33 years after the original diagnosis.

Gonadoblastomas frequently contain calcifications that can be detected by plain radiography of the pelvis. Women who have gonadoblastomas often have ambiguous genitalia. The tumors are usually small and, in one-third of affected women, bilateral.

The malignant potential of immature teratomas correlates with the degree of immature or embryonic tissue present. The presence of choriocarcinoma can be determined histologically as well as by HCG assays. The presence of choriocarcinoma in an immature teratoma worsens the prognosis.

204-207. The answers are: 204-B, 205-C, 206-D, 207-A. *(Novak, ed 7. pp 375-382, 427-431, 450-456, 469-476.)* Granulosa cell tumors show considerable microscopic variation. In most instances constituent cells resemble granulosa cells; and Call-Exner bodies, which are small liquefied cysts common in granulosa cells, may be observed in the better-differentiated forms of the tumor.

Arrhenoblastomas are malignant, masculinizing ovarian tumors. Testicular structures may be present (in the accompanying micrograph, testicular-like tubules can be observed). Reinke crystalloids also are often noted.

Benign cystic teratomas are the most common type of ovarian teratoma. The presence of sebaceous glandular elements are common; bone, cartilage, hair follicles, and skin also are frequently encountered.

Mucinous cystadenomas are characterized by the presence of the familiar, columnar, mucin-producing cells lining the cyst cavity. No evidence of malignancy typically is found.

Endocrinology and Infertility

Alan H. DeCherney

DIRECTIONS: Each question below contains five suggested answers. Choose the **one best** response to each question.

208. A 46-year-old woman presents with depression, urinary urgency, night sweats, and headaches. On examination she is found to be anovulatory. The most likely diagnosis is

(A) psychosomatic disorder
(B) manic depression
(C) urinary-tract infection
(D) tuberculosis with renal involvement
(E) menopause

209. A 35-year-old woman presents with hypotension, cold intolerance, amenorrhea, waxy skin with multiple fine wrinkles, loss of axillary and pubic hair, and loss of skin pigmentation. Her urine sodium levels are normal. The most likely diagnosis is

(A) hypothyroidism
(B) Addison's disease
(C) panhypopituitarism
(D) malignant melanoma
(E) diabetes insipidus

210. A 22-year-old woman, gravida 0, has oligomenorrhea, hirsutism, and fertility problems. Neither muscle mass nor clitoral size is increased. Elevated androgen-production rates are found, and ovarian biopsy shows stromal hyperplasia and follicular cells at all stages of development. The most likely diagnosis is

(A) Turner's syndrome
(B) Stein-Leventhal syndrome
(C) Kallman's syndrome
(D) Reifenstein's syndrome
(E) adrenogenital syndrome

211. In the testis, which of the following can be **directly** influenced by luteinizing hormone (LH)?

(A) Leydig cells
(B) Sertoli cells
(C) Leydig cells and Sertoli cells
(D) Leydig cells and seminiferous tubules
(E) Sertoli cells and seminiferous tubules

212. A 55-year-old woman who, ten years earlier, had a total abdominal hysterectomy and bilateral salpingo-oophorectomy for moderate endometriosis, now complains of debilitating hot flashes and depression. The most appropriate therapy for this woman would be

(A) observation
(B) combined birth-control pills
(C) conjugated estrogens (Premarin), 1.25 mg daily for 21 days every month
(D) chlorpromazine (Thorazine), 200 mg daily
(E) exploratory laparotomy

213. A 39-year-old woman, gravida 2, para 2, who complains of pelvic pain, is found on laparoscopy to have extensive endometriosis. She does not want more children. The most appropriate treatment would be

(A) danazol
(B) oral contraceptives
(C) radical hysterectomy (Wertheim's operation)
(D) total abdominal hysterectomy with conservation of uninvolved ovaries
(E) total abdominal hysterectomy and bilateral salpingo-oophorectomy

214. Which of the following statements about the derivation of urinary testosterone in men is true?

(A) One-hundred percent is testicular in origin
(B) Ninety-five percent is derived from the testes and five percent from the adrenal glands
(C) Fifty percent is derived from the testes and fifty percent from the adrenal glands
(D) One-hundred percent is adrenal in origin
(E) Its derivation cannot be accurately determined

215. In pituitary failure, the usual order of appearance of clinical deficiencies of the tropic hormones is

(A) somatotropin, thyrotropin, corticotropin, prolactin, gonadotropin
(B) thyrotropin, corticotropin, prolactin, gonadotropin, somatotropin
(C) corticotropin, prolactin, gonadotropin, somatotropin, thyrotropin
(D) prolactin, gonadotropin, somatotropin, thyrotropin, corticotropin
(E) gonadotropin, somatotropin, thyrotropin, corticotropin, prolactin

216. The diaphragma sellae is composed of

(A) a reflection of the dura mater
(B) a reflection of the pia mater
(C) a reflection of the arachnoid membrane
(D) cranial bones
(E) pituitary blood vessels

217. Which of the following statements about the human pituitary gland is true?

(A) Three-fourths of its weight is in the posterior portion, one-fourth in the anterior
(B) It has a prominent pars intermedia
(C) Part of it arises embryologically from Rathke's pouch
(D) It is nonfunctional in the fetus until the third trimester
(E) It has an active anastomotic blood supply connecting the anterior and posterior portions

218. Which of the following steps in the mechanism of action of corticotropin (ACTH) is INCORRECT?

(A) ACTH is bound by specific surface receptors on the adrenal cortical cell
(B) In the presence of magnesium, adenylcyclase is activated and the intracellular concentration of cyclic AMP increases
(C) Cyclic AMP phosphorylates key enzymes
(D) Key enzymes facilitate the conversion of cholesterol to pregnenolone
(E) Synthesis of new proteins also occurs and increases adrenal weight

219. The management of girls who have idiopathic precocious puberty includes

(A) progestin therapy
(B) estrogen therapy
(C) androgen therapy
(D) pelvic irradiation
(E) laparoscopy

220. Which of the following statements about prolactin is true?

(A) It potentiates the action of testosterone in men
(B) It causes an unprimed mammary gland to secrete milk
(C) It acts through the release of thyrotropin to produce milk secretion
(D) It promotes nesting behavior in some species of birds
(E) It has significant luteotrophic properties in women

221. Which of the following statements about precocious puberty in girls is true?

(A) It is rarely idiopathic
(B) It often is heralded by a growth spurt
(C) Menarche is usually the first symptom
(D) Fertility tests are crucial for affected girls
(E) True sexual precocity cannot stem from neoplastic causes

222. If the aim of artificial insemination is to inseminate a woman at the exact time of ovulation, the best time for insemination, relative to the measured LH peak, would be

(A) 12 to 24 hours before the LH peak
(B) at the peak
(C) 2 to 5 hours after the peak
(D) 16 to 24 hours after the peak
(E) 25 to 48 hours after the peak

223. The manufacture of ethinyl estradiol was an important breakthrough in the development of oral contraceptives, because the agent was discovered to be

(A) an especially effective contraceptive
(B) orally active
(C) half as potent as diethylstilbestrol
(D) the endogenously active form of estrogen
(E) the compound making development of "minipills" possible

224. The use of combined birth-control pills is absolutely contraindicated in women who have all of the following EXCEPT

(A) sickle cell anemia
(B) diabetes
(C) cholestatic liver disease
(D) atrial fibrillation
(E) history of thromboemboli

225. The usual order of appearance of the signs of normal puberty is

(A) axillary hair, breast buds, pubic hair, menarche
(B) breast buds, axillary hair, pubic hair, menarche
(C) breast buds, pubic hair, axillary hair, menarche
(D) pubic hair, menarche, breast buds, axillary hair
(E) pubic hair, breast buds, menarche, axillary hair

226. A 28-year-old woman has galactorrhea and amenorrhea. Pertinent laboratory studies reveal normal levels of follicle-stimulating hormone (FSH) and LH but a prolactin level of 35 ng/ml (normal: less than 20 ng/ml); tomograms of the sella show no erosion, and a pneumoencephalogram also is read as normal. Treatment of this woman, who has no desire for further pregnancy, should include

(A) L-dopa
(B) thorazine
(C) brom-ergotryptine
(D) neurosurgery
(E) pituitary irradiation

227. Amenorrhea can be associated with all of the following EXCEPT

(A) hematometra
(B) uterus didelphys
(C) testicular feminization
(D) Turner's syndrome
(E) Sheehan's syndrome

228. The hormone primarily responsible for production of sex steroids is

(A) FSH
(B) LH
(C) ACTH
(D) thyroid-stimulating hormone (TSH)
(E) prolactin

229. A 19-year-old man is seen because of late onset of puberty. The laboratory reports the man has azoospermia; and physical and historical findings indicate that he also has a poorly developed sense of smell. The most likely diagnosis is

(A) panhypopituitarism
(B) Reifenstein's syndrome
(C) Klinefelter's syndrome
(D) Kallman's syndrome
(E) Turner's syndrome

230. If a man received a severe thermal trauma to his testes, his sperm count, which was previously normal, would become depressed in about

(A) 1 day
(B) 7 days
(C) 30 days
(D) 75 days
(E) 100 days

231. The Sertoli-cell-only syndrome is characterized by

(A) increased FSH levels
(B) increased LH levels
(C) increased FSH and LH levels
(D) decreased FSH and LH levels
(E) normal FSH and LH levels

DIRECTIONS: Each question below contains four suggested answers of which **one** or **more** is correct. Choose the answer:

A	if	**1, 2, and 3**	are correct
B	if	**1 and 3**	are correct
C	if	**2 and 4**	are correct
D	if	**4**	is correct
E	if	**1, 2, 3, and 4**	are correct

232. Physiologic processes that are estrogen-dependent in women include which of the following?

(1) Menses
(2) Vaginal cornification
(3) Appearance of axillary hair
(4) Cervical mucus formation

233. Which of the following statements concerning early development of the ovary are true?

(1) Germ cells in the fetal ovary migrated from the yolk sac
(2) The maximum population of oogonia is reached at about 20 weeks gestation
(3) The fetal ovary is indistinguishable from the fetal testis until the sixth week of gestation
(4) The wolffian system is prominent before the müllerian system

234. Which of the following organs CANNOT synthesize cholesterol from acetate?

(1) Ovary
(2) Adrenal gland
(3) Testis
(4) Placenta

235. Waning estrogen levels in perimenopausal women can produce which of the following?

(1) Vasomotor instability
(2) Atrophic vaginitis
(3) Decreased libido
(4) Osteoporosis

236. The luteal phase of the menstrual cycle primarily involves which of the following?

(1) Δ^4-3-Ketone pathway
(2) Δ^5-3β-Hydroxy pathway
(3) Granulosa cells
(4) Theca cells

237. Rising estradiol levels can have which of the following hormonal effects?

(1) Suppression of LH
(2) Stimulation of LH
(3) Suppression of FSH
(4) Stimulation of FSH

238. Estrogen administration is considered definitely advantageous in the treatment of perimenopausal women who have

(1) emotional reactions
(2) vasomotor reactions
(3) osteoporosis
(4) atherosclerosis

239. Side effects of estrogen replacement therapy include which of the following?

(1) Dyspareunia
(2) Edema
(3) Weight loss
(4) Breast tenderness

240. The use of estrogen replacement therapy may be hazardous, if not expressly contraindicated, for women who have

(1) impaired hepatic function
(2) thromboembolic disorders
(3) vaginal bleeding
(4) estrogen-dependent tumors

241. Retrograde menstruation is the most accepted explanation of the etiology of endometriosis. Which of the following statements may be cited as evidence for this theory?

(1) Inversion of the cervix of a monkey into the peritoneal cavity can cause endometriosis
(2) Endometrial tissue can be cultured successfully
(3) Menstrual blood can come from the ends of the fallopian tubes of some women
(4) Endometrial glands can arise from coelomic epithelium

242. An 18-year-old woman has primary amenorrhea. Her growth and development have been normal. Work-up of this woman should include

(1) serum FSH and LH levels
(2) karyotype
(3) serum prolactin levels
(4) an endometrial biopsy

243. The physiologic effects of endogenous oxytocin include

(1) relaxation of vascular smooth muscles
(2) initiation of milk production
(3) a marked antidiuretic-hormone effect
(4) stimulation of uterine contractions

244. Signs or symptoms commonly associated with anorexia nervosa but NOT with hypopituitarism are

(1) marked wasting
(2) loss of axillary and pubic hair
(3) elevated levels of human growth hormone
(4) decreased thyroid activity

245. Mammary-gland development is a common feature of patients who have

(1) testicular feminization
(2) Reifenstein's syndrome
(3) Klinefelter's syndrome
(4) Turner's syndrome

246. The causes of panhypopituitarism include

(1) postpartum hemorrhage
(2) Hand-Schüller-Christian disease
(3) temporal arteritis
(4) empty-sella syndrome

SUMMARY OF DIRECTIONS

A	B	C	D	E
1, 2, 3 only	1, 3 only	2, 4 only	4 only	All are correct

247. Which of the following statements about the morphology and function of sex chromosomes are true?

(1) Testicular development does not occur in XXY individuals
(2) The Y chromosome is of equal size in all men
(3) Individuals who have a 45,YO karyotype undergo late-onset puberty
(4) The karyotype 46,XX has been discovered in phenotypic males

248. Characteristics of the gonadotropins (FSH and LH) include

(1) stimulation of the production of primordial follicles
(2) stimulation of the production of estrogen by thecal cells
(3) stimulation of the production of spermatozoa and testosterone in men who have hypopituitarism
(4) a glycoprotein structure

249. Which of the following hormones have overlapping structural compositions and similar biologic modes of action?

(1) Prolactin
(2) Growth hormone
(3) Chorionic somatomammotropin
(4) Thyrotropin

250. Which of the following compounds can decrease prolactin secretion?

(1) Phenothiozines
(2) Alpha-methyldopa
(3) Serotonin
(4) Levodopa

251. A 26-year-old woman, who comes to your office to renew her supply of birth-control pills, has mild hypertension, truncal obesity, and acne. Laboratory evaluation reveals that her serum levels of free cortisol are increased; this increase could be due to which of the following reasons?

(1) Cushing's disease
(2) Displacement of cortisol from transcortin by progesterone
(3) Estrogen-related interference of the liver's ability to metabolize cortisol
(4) An increase in ACTH production caused by ingestion of birth-control pills

252. Endocrine causes of short stature in young women include

(1) hypothyroidism
(2) adrenal hyperplasia
(3) Cushing's disease
(4) Turner's syndrome

253. Progestational agents in birth-control pills have which of the following actions?

(1) Inhibition of secretion of hypothalamic releasing factor
(2) Endometrial decidualization
(3) Thickening of cervical mucus
(4) Prevention of irregular menses

254. Which of the following statements about postpartum lactation are true?

(1) Breast engorgement occurs during the first postpartum day
(2) Only colostrum is produced at the time of delivery
(3) Prolactin levels rise steadily after delivery and peak at one month postpartum
(4) Oxytocin is not crucial for the production of milk

255. In the mother, suckling leads to which of the following?

(1) Synthesis of oxytocin
(2) Inhibition of prolactin inhibitory factor
(3) Decrease of hypothalamic dopamine
(4) Release of luteinizing-hormone releasing factor

256. Which of the following are types of endometrial dysfunctional bleeding?

(1) Estrogen breakthrough bleeding
(2) Estrogen withdrawal bleeding
(3) Progesterone breakthrough bleeding
(4) Progesterone withdrawal bleeding

257. Asherman's syndrome is characterized by which of the following?

(1) Biphasic basal body temperatures
(2) Diagnosis by endometrial biopsy
(3) Amenorrhea
(4) Remission after removal of an intrauterine device

DIRECTIONS: The groups of questions below consist of lettered choices followed by several numbered items. For each numbered item select the **one** lettered choice with which it is **most** closely associated. Each lettered choice may be used once, more than once, or not at all.

Questions 258-262

For each description that follows, select the phase of the ovulatory cycle with which it most likely is associated.

(A) Proliferative phase
(B) Secretory phase
(C) Preparation-for-implantation phase
(D) Endometrial-breakdown phase
(E) Menstrual-endometrium phase

258. Growth of endometrial components in an endometrium of fixed height

259. Significant glandular mitosis

260. Three distinct endometrial zones

261. "Reinflation" of the stroma

262. Alternating vasodilatation and vasoconstriction of spiral arterioles

Questions 263-268

For each description that follows, select the type of sexual precocity with which it most likely is associated.

(A) True sexual precocity
(B) Incomplete sexual precocity
(C) Isosexual precocious pseudopuberty
(D) Heterosexual precocious pseudopuberty
(E) Precocity due to gonadotropin-producing tumors

263. Can be associated with a positive pregnancy test in nonpregnant girls

264. Defined by the presence of virilizing signs in girls

265. Characterized by the presence of premature adrenarche, pubarche, or thelarche

266. Can arise from cranial tumors or hypothyroidism

267. Stems from premature activation of the hypothalamus-pituitary system

268. Frequently caused by ovarian tumors

Questions 269-273

For each description that follows, select the pharmacologic agent with which it is most likely to be associated.

(A) Ethinyl estradiol
(B) Mestranol
(C) Norethindrone
(D) Clomiphene
(E) Medroxyprogesterone acetate

269. The estrogen component of Enovid, Norinyl, and Ortho-Novum

270. The progestin component of most oral contraceptives

271. Associated with production of benign breast tumors in dogs

272. Commercially marketed as Provera

273. An antiestrogenic agent

Questions 274-277

For each of the following loci, select the appropriate position in the cholesterol molecule pictured below.

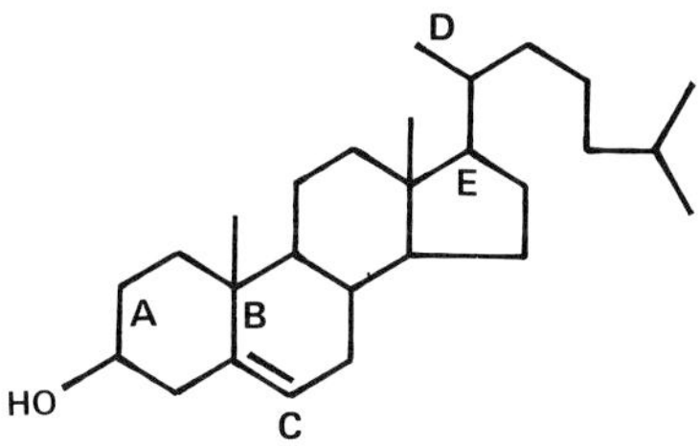

274. 6 position

275. 10 position

276. 17 position

277. 21 position

Questions 278-282

Match the following.

(A) Adenylcyclase
(B) 5α-Reductase
(C) 17β-Hydroxylase
(D) 20-Hydroxylase
(E) 21-Dehydroxylase

278. Is activated by LH

279. Converts androstenedione to testosterone

280. Converts testosterone to dihydrotestosterone

281. Catalyzes the first step in the production of hormonal steroids from cholesterol

282. Congenital deficiency causes massive adrenal enlargement, is associated with poor survival of affected infants, and can lead to formation of female genitalia in genotypically male infants

Questions 283-286

For each case history that follows, select the type of menstrual bleeding with which it most likely is associated.

(A) Progesterone breakthrough bleeding
(B) Progesterone withdrawal bleeding
(C) Estrogen breakthrough bleeding
(D) Estrogen withdrawal bleeding
(E) None of the above

283. A 24-year-old nulligravid woman is being evaluated for infertility. Her cycles are irregular, lasting from 30 to 90 days. Menstrual flow is usually heavy. She also has increasing hirsutism and obesity

284. A 55-year-old woman, three years postmenopause, is bothered by hot flashes. Her doctor orders conjugated estrogens (Premarin), 1.25 mg daily for 21 of 28 days. On the fourth month of Premarin therapy, the woman has heavy menstrual flow from the 25th to the 28th day

285. An 18-year-old woman complains of severe dysmenorrhea. She has regular periods every 28 days, with light flow on the first day, heavy flow on the second and third days, and light spotting on the fourth day

286. A 33-year-old woman is placed on one of the newer low-dose birth-control pills. Two weeks later, having taken nine of the birth-control pills, she calls your office because she has begun to have menstrual flow

Questions 287-291

Match the following.

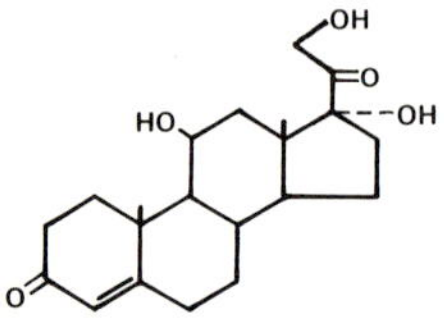

Cortisol
A

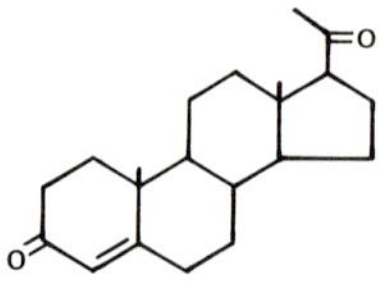

Progesterone
B

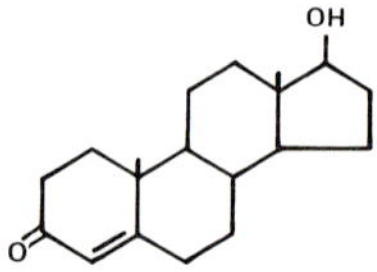

Testosterone
C

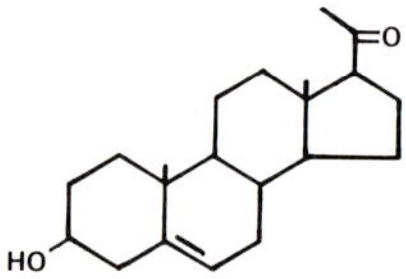

Δ^5-Pregnenolone
D

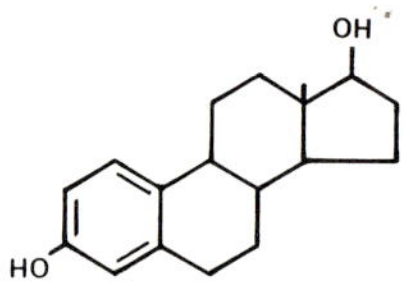

Estradiol-17β
E

287. Produced by Leydig cells

288. Can be detected by the Porter-Silber reaction

289. Secreted by arrhenoblastomas

290. An essential precursor in the theca-interna production of estrogen

291. An essential precursor in the granulosa-cell production of estrogen

Endocrinology and Infertility

Answers

208. The answer is E. *(Speroff, pp 49-50.)* The symptoms described in the question are common symptoms of menopause. They all result primarily from estrogen withdrawal, and most can be reversed by estrogen therapy. "Climacteric" is actually a better word for this complex of symptoms, because the menopause is technically the instant at which menses cease.

209. The answer is C. *(Williams, ed 5. pp 55-59.)* The most likely diagnosis in the woman described in the question is panhypopituitarism. The associated hypotension results from a decrease in cortisone production, which is caused by a lack of corticotropin. Because the adrenal glands still maintain the ability to produce aldosterone, sodium levels are usually unchanged. Cold intolerance, amenorrhea, and changes in skin appearance and pigmentation are frequent signs of hypopituitarism. A patient who has hypothyroidism generally would present with different symptoms from those described, although cold intolerance may be encountered. A patient with Addison's disease would not be able to maintain body sodium. Malignant melanoma causes none of the presenting features described; and although diabetes insipidus may be a symptom of hypopituitarism, it too does not cause the described symptomatology.

210. The answer is B. *(Speroff, pp 60-63.)* Because the woman described in the question is able to menstruate, she clearly does not have either Turner's or Reifenstein's syndrome. Kallman's syndrome is hypogonadotropic amenorrhea; women who have this disease rarely have increased androgen-production rates. The differential diagnosis in the case rests then between Stein-Leventhal syndrome and the adrenogenital syndrome. Women who have adrenogenital syndrome are virilized and have a muscular physique, cliteromegaly, and temporal recession of hair. That this patient shows only hirsutism indicates that the diagnosis is Stein-Leventhal syndrome.

211. The answer is A. *(Williams, ed 5. pp 324-329.)* In the testis, Leydig cells produce testosterone, Sertoli cells primarily provide structural support and nutrition, and seminiferous tubules produce sperm. Leydig cells are under the influence of luteinizing hormone (LH) in a negative-feedback relationship. Testosterone produced by Leydig cells regulates spermatogenesis; therefore, seminiferous tubules are indirectly affected by LH secretion.

212. The answer is C. *(Speroff, pp 84, 202.)* The woman described in the question is having severe menopausal symptoms and should be treated with conjugated estrogens (Premarin), 1.25 mg daily, in a cyclic fashion. Despite common myths, many studies have shown that estrogen does not exacerbate old endometriotic lesions. Cyclic combined birth-control pills, however, would not be recommended for this woman's treatment, because they possibly could stimulate old endometrial implants (progesterone seems to be necessary for stimulation). Exploratory laparotomy is not indicated for this patient and would have no beneficial effect. Similarly, use of chlorpromazine (Thorazine), a major tranquilizer, also is not indicated.

213. The answer is E. *(Speroff, pp 200-202.)* Because the woman described does not want more children, the definitive and only curative procedure would be a total abdominal hysterectomy and bilateral salpingo-oophorectomy. Retaining any ovarian tissue would be contraindicated, because the constant production of hormone would stimulate the endometrial implants not detected during the original surgery and thus would cause the patient's symptoms to recur. The use of danazol, an antigonadotropin, or oral contraceptives to treat the woman described would only suppress and decidualize the endometrial implants. Both treatments are temporary measures only.

214. The answer is B. *(Williams, ed 5. p 327.)* Ninety-five percent of urinary testosterone is derived from the testes. The adrenal gland accounts for the other 5 percent by producing Δ^4-andostenedione, which the liver converts to testosterone glucuronide.

215. The answer is E. *(Williams, ed 5. p 56.)* In pituitary failure, the tropic hormones usually disappear in the following order: gonadotropin, somatotropin, thyrotropin, corticotropin, and prolactin. When all the tropic hormones are gone, the diagnosis of pituitary failure is easy; however, in the evaluation of possible incipient pituitary failure, the sequential disappearance of these hormones can be an important diagnostic clue. Thus, a woman who develops amenorrhea followed by symptoms of thyroid dysfunction should be suspected of having pituitary failure.

216. The answer is A. *(Williams, ed 5. p 31.)* The diaphragma sellae is a reflection of the dura mater and separates the pituitary gland from the other cranial contents. The stalk of and the blood vessels to the pituitary gland go through the diaphragma sellae.

217. The answer is C. *(Williams, ed 5. pp 31-32.)* The human pituitary gland arises in part from Rathke's pouch, an ectodermal evagination. Three-fourths of the weight of the human pituitary gland is in the anterior portion and one-fourth in the posterior. The fetal gland begins to function about the twelfth week of gestation, as proven by the isolation at this stage of corticotropin and thyrotropin. There is little anastomotic blood flow between the anterior pituitary and posterior pituitary. In the human pituitary gland, the pars intermedia is nearly nonexistent.

218. The answer is B. *(Williams, ed 5. p 38.)* Corticotropin (ACTH) binds to specific cell-surface receptors in the adrenal cortex and is concentrated from the plasma. The combined action of ACTH and calcium stimulates adenylcyclase to catalyze production of cyclic AMP, which in turn causes enzyme phosphorylation. These enzymes convert precursors to active hormones; cholesterol, for example, is converted enzymatically to pregnenolone. Cyclic AMP also induces synthesis of RNA, which in turn stimulates protein synthesis; as a result, adrenal weight is increased.

219. The answer is A. *(Speroff, p 141.)* Progestin therapy is the treatment of choice for girls who have idiopathic precocious puberty. Although progestins cannot cause pubic hair to disappear, they can stop future growth, arrest breast development, and, most important, cause bone growth to decelerate, thus preventing early epiphyseal closure. Progestin treatment should be stopped when bone age equals chronologic age. Estrogen therapy is contraindicated, because it can only exacerbate symptoms of precocity and result in short stature. Laparoscopy is not indicated, because most causes of precocious puberty can eventually be determined without surgery.

220. The answer is D. *(Williams, ed 5. pp 46-47.)* Prolactin's only known function in humans is the stimulation of lactation. In order for prolactin to initiate milk production, the mammary glands must be primed with estrogen, progesterone, cortisol, and insulin; it has no effect on the unprimed breast. Prolactin also has no effect on the release of thyrotropin, and no known interaction between the two hormones exists. Luteotrophic effects of prolactin have never been documented in women, and the hormone has no established role in men. Prolactin can induce behavioral changes, including the promotion of nesting behavior, in some species of birds.

221. **The answer is B.** *(Speroff, p 137.)* Precocious puberty is usually heralded by an earlier-than-expected growth spurt. Although it most commonly is idiopathic or constitutional, sexual precocity, even if accompanied by ovulation and progesterone production, can be brought on by certain disease states, such as tumors of the ovary or central nervous system. Menarche may appear as the initial symptom of precocious puberty; more often, however, it is a late symptom, depending on the production of high levels of gonadotropins over a period of time. Tests for fertility, such as progesterone assays, usually are not necessary.

222. **The answer is D.** *(Speroff, p 35.)* Because ovulation occurs 16 to 24 hours after the LH peak, this is the best time to artificially inseminate a woman. An ovum can be fertilized at any time during approximately the first 12 hours after ovulation.

223. **The answer is B.** *(Goodman, ed 5. pp 1431, 1442-1443. Speroff, p 152.)* An ethinyl group added at the 17 position makes ethinyl estradiol a very potent, orally active estrogen. Until this discovery in 1938, no orally effective estrogen had been manufactured. The contraceptive properties of ethinyl estradiol are not significantly different from other estrogens. Ethinyl estradiol, which is up to 25 times as potent as diethylstilbestrol, is not a constituent of "minipill" birth-control pills.

224. **The answer is B.** *(Speroff, pp 162-167.)* Sickle cell anemia, atrial fibrillation, and previous pulmonary embolus are contraindications to the use of birth-control pills, because clotting is enhanced by increased levels of fibrinogen. It also has been shown that oral contraceptives markedly increase cholestasis in women who are sensitive to this effect of estrogen; this cholestasis resembles cholestasic jaundice of pregnancy. Although diabetes might be made worse in diabetic women taking birth-control pills, the value of effective contraception may outweigh the pills' negative effects; for these women, an increase in their insulin dose may be a satisfactory precaution. The use of oral contraceptives, however, is not recommended for diabetic women who do not take insulin but who would require it once oral contraceptive therapy has begun.

225. **The answer is C.** *(Speroff, p 135.)* The appearance of breast buds is dependent on early estrogen production and is usually the first sign of puberty. Increased production of androgens causes the development of pubic hair and, about two years later, axillary hair. Menarche then occurs, usually after the growth spurt has peaked.

226. The answer is C. *(Speroff, p 110.)* Ergot alkaloids, such as brom-ergotryptine, would be effective treatment for the woman described in the question, because they directly inhibit pituitary prolactin release. L-Dopa is converted in the hypothalamus to dopamine, which suppresses the production of prolactin inhibitory factor and thus increases the release of prolactin. Administration of chlorpromazine (Thorazine), which inhibits the production of prolactin inhibitory factor, would exacerbate the woman's galactorrhea. Neurosurgery or radiation therapy are not indicated for this woman, because no demonstrable tumor has been shown; from her symptoms, however, the possibility that a tumor may emerge in the future cannot be ruled out.

227. The answer is B. *(Speroff, pp 78-83.)* Didelphia (double uterus) develops due to failure of müllerian structures to fuse in the midline. The endometrium is normal, and menstruation usually occurs from both uteri and both cervices. Hematometra, which is the accumulation of blood in the uterus, results from cervical stenosis; no blood flows out of the cervix, although the endometrium has normal shedding. Individuals who have testicular feminization have no uterus, thus making menstruation impossible. Women who have Turner's syndrome have nonfunctional ovaries; their amenorrhea is of the hypergonadotropic, hypoestrogenic variety. Certain forms of Turner's syndrome mosaicisms, however, are associated with normal menstruation. Amenorrhea in Sheehan's syndrome is caused by the absence of FSH and LH production by the pituitary gland. Hence, the ovaries are not stimulated to produce estrogen and, as a result, normal menstruation does not occur.

228. The answer is B. *(Speroff, pp 16-17.)* FSH is responsible for spermatocyte production and ovum maturation, and LH is primarily responsible for production of hormones (e.g., the production of progesterone by the granulosa cells of the ovary). Prolactin, ACTH, and TSH have no known role in sex-steroid production. LH probably is responsible for the actual act of ovulation and may activate cholesterol esterase, which catalyzes production of cholesterol (the precursor of steroids and, therefore, of the sex steroids) and free fatty acids (prostaglandin precursors).

229. The answer is D. *(Williams, ed 5. pp 60-61.)* The man described in the question has Kallman's syndrome, which is a combination of hypogonadotropic eunuchoidism and hyposmia (an abnormally decreased sense of smell). Whether these two symptoms share a common etiology is not known. Panhypopituitarism and Reifenstein's and Klinefelter's syndromes all can lead to hypogonadism, but none are associated with abnormalities in the sense of smell. Turner's syndrome is gonadal dysgenesis in an individual who has a 45,XO karyotype.

230. The answer is D. *(Williams, ed 5. p 325.)* Severe trauma to the testes, such as that caused by cold or heat, can inhibit the development of sperm. Depression in the sperm count usually appears in about 75 days, the length of time in which an immature spermatid develops into a spermatozoon. Either oligospermia or azoospermia can result.

231. The answer is A. *(Williams, ed 5. pp 328-329.)* The Sertoli-cell-only syndrome is characterized by an increase in FSH levels; LH levels remain normal. There are two major theories to explain how the testis controls FSH production. One is the "inhibin" theory, in which the germinal epithelium is thought to produce a water-soluble, nonsteroid substance that regulates FSH secretion. The other theory states that Sertoli cells secrete a steroid, possibly Δ^5-pregnenolone, that controls FSH production. In a testis containing only Sertoli cells, there would be no regulation on, hence no negative feedback of, FSH; FSH levels therefore would be elevated.

232. The answer is E (all). *(Speroff, p 45.)* The presence of estrogen in a pubertal woman stimulates the formation of secondary sex characteristics, including development of breasts, appearance of axillary hair, production of cervical mucus, and vaginal cornification. As estrogen levels increase, menses begins and ovulation is maintained for several decades. Decreasing levels of estrogen lower the frequency of ovulation, eventually leading to the menopause.

233. The answer is A (1, 2, 3). *(Speroff, pp 39-42.)* The early fetal ovary is an undeveloped gonad, composed of connective tissue of mesenchymal origin and germ cells that have migrated from the yolk sac during a five-week period. Until about the first six weeks of gestation have elapsed, the primitive ovary is indistinguishable from the primitive testis. The müllerian duct system (which develops into the uterus and other female reproductive structures) is present until 12 weeks gestation, when, if a testicular gonad is present, the wolffian system develops and the müllerian system disappears. The number of oogonia decreases from about 7 million at 20 weeks gestation to about 300,000 at puberty.

234. The answer is D (4). *(Speroff, p 7.)* The conversion of acetate to cholesterol and, hence, to all the other steroid hormones can occur in the ovary, testis, and adrenal gland. The placenta, however, lacks the essential enzyme systems to perform this synthesis. Therefore, cholesterol, the basic building block in the synthesis of steroid hormones, must be supplied to the placenta.

235. The answer is E (all). *(Speroff, p 49.)* In menopausal and postmenopausal women, waning estrogen levels can produce atrophic vaginitis, decreased libido, vasomotor instability, osteoporosis, and psychological symptoms (including depression and anxiety). Vasomotor instability causes the familiar hot flashes of menopausal women. These responses may be due to an unstable relationship, caused by decreased estrogen levels, between the autonomic nervous system and hypothalamus.

236. The answer is B (1, 3). *(Speroff, p 43.)* In the luteal phase of the menstrual cycle, granulosa cells produce estrogen by way of the Δ^4-3-ketone pathway, in which progesterone is a precursor. Theca cells in the follicular phase of the menstrual cycle manufacture estrogen by the Δ^5-3β-hydroxy pathway; pregnenolone, dehydroepiandrosterone, and estradiol—but not progesterone—are essential precursors of this pathway.

237. The answer is A (1, 2, 3). *(Speroff, pp 32-33.)* Estradiol has a negative-feedback relationship with follicle-stimulating hormone (FSH) and both a negative-feedback and positive-feedback relationship with LH. Rising estradiol levels suppress the production of FSH and LH. As estradiol levels continue to increase, however, LH levels begin to rise. Negative feedback (suppression of LH and FSH production) is mediated by estradiol effects on the hypothalamus and pituitary gland; positive feedback (increase in LH) also is controlled by hypothalamic centers.

238. The answer is A (1, 2, 3). *(Speroff, pp 52-53.)* There is good evidence that estrogen reduces anxiety, depression, and other emotional reactions that can accompany menopause. Estrogens also are helpful in retarding osteoporosis, although their use cannot replace the calcium that already has been lost. The clearest response to estrogen therapy is by the autonomic nervous system; relief from vasomotor reactions, such as hot flashes, by the use of estrogens is significant. The usefulness of estrogen therapy relative to atherosclerosis is, at present, undetermined. Although atherosclerosis seems to occur more frequently in women who have premature menopause, administration of estrogens does not have clear therapeutic or prophylactic effects in postmenopausal women.

239. The answer is C (2, 4). *(Speroff, pp 51-53.)* Side effects of estrogen replacement therapy can include edema, weight gain, increased vaginal bleeding, and breast tenderness. Development of these side effects usually occurs in conjunction with inappropriately high doses of estrogen. Dyspareunia, along with vaginitis, dysuria, pruritus, and other symptoms, is associated with decreased levels of estrogen.

240. The answer is E (all). *(Speroff, p 52.)* The use of estrogen replacement therapy can be deleterious for women who are bleeding or who have thromboembolic symptoms. Because the liver is influenced significantly by estrogens, which can affect the function of hepatic cell enzymes and production of lipids and lipoproteins, the effects of hepatic impairment can be exacerbated by estrogen therapy. The existence of estrogen-dependent tumors is a contraindication to estrogen use.

241. The answer is A (1, 2, 3). *(Speroff, p 199.)* Retrograde menstruation is currently believed to be a major cause of endometriosis. Supporting this belief are the following findings: inversion of the uterine cervix into the peritoneal cavity can cause a monkey to develop endometriosis; endometrial tissue is viable outside the uterus; and blood can issue from the ends of the fallopian tubes of some women during menstruation. The fact that endometrial implants can occur in the lung implies that lymphatic or vascular routes of spread of the disease also are possible. Another theory of the etiology of endometriosis entails the conversion of coelomic epithelium into glands resembling those of the endometrium.

242. The answer is A (1, 2, 3). *(Speroff, pp 75-78.)* In the work-up of primary amenorrhea, serum FSH and LH determinations can help to establish whether a woman has primary pituitary failure. A karyotype is important to rule out a genetic etiology, such as Turner's syndrome. Determination of serum prolactin levels is now practicable and becoming more popular in the work-up of amenorrhea. (Prolactin is elevated in many of the pituitary microadenomas causing amenorrhea.) An endometrial biopsy in the work-up of primary amenorrhea is of no value whatsoever.

243. The answer is D (4). *(Williams, ed 5. p 92.)* Oxytocin causes uterine contractions by an as yet unknown mechanism. It does not cause milk production, which is dependent on the presence of insulin, cortisone, estrogen, progesterone, and prolactin; rather, oxytocin stimulates milk ejection by causing myoepithelial cells to contract. Endogenous oxytocin has an extremely mild antidiuretic-hormone effect. When large pharmacologic doses of oxytocin are administered, the potential for antidiuresis increases and smooth-muscle relaxation, causing transient hypotension, can occur.

244. The answer is B (1, 3). *(Thorn, ed 8. p 208. Williams, ed 5. p 58.)* Patients who have anorexia nervosa show a striking loss of body mass on physical examination; patients who have panhypopituitarism, however, show marked wasting only infrequently. Axillary and pubic hair are not lost in patients affected by anorexia nervosa, because circulating steroid levels are maintained. Steroid levels in panhypopituitarism, on the other hand, are low, causing loss of axillary and pubic hair. In panhypopituitarism, the human growth hormone level is extremely low and thyroid activity is decreased significantly; these values are either normal or elevated in anorectic individuals.

245. The answer is A (1, 2, 3). *(Williams, ed 5. pp 449-459, 484-487.)* The degree of mammary-gland development depends on the relationship between estrogen and androgen production and utilization. Development of mammary tissue is significant in individuals who have testicular feminization, in which peripheral testosterone use is very low; Reifenstein's syndrome, in which serum testosterone levels are reduced; or Klinefelter's syndrome, in which testosterone production is decreased but estrogen production remains normal or near normal. On the other hand, mammary-gland development is not characteristic of Turner's syndrome patients, who produce no androgen and very little estrogen.

246. The answer is E (all). *(Williams, ed 5. p 56.)* Postpartum panhypopituitarism is caused by hemorrhage in and subsequent necrosis of the pituitary gland, which is enlarged during pregnancy. Temporal arteritis and sickle cell anemia lead to panhypopituitarism by causing chronic vascular insufficiency of the pituitary gland. Hand-Schüller-Christian disease causes panhypopituitarism as a result of the infiltration of the gland by cholesterol-laden histiocytes. In the empty-sella syndrome, the pituitary gland becomes compressed within the sella. The pressure eventually necroses the tissue, and the gland becomes nonfunctional.

247. The answer is D (4). *(Williams, ed 5. p 439.)* The presence of a Y chromosome, which can vary in size among men, is necessary for testicular development to occur; individuals who have a 47,XXY karyotype, therefore, will undergo some degree of testicular growth. The development of female genitalia is mediated by the second X chromosome, although this effect is less direct than that of the Y chromosome on male genital development. The YO genetic pattern is a lethal one, with no incidences of viable affected fetuses reported. Although the 46,XX karyotype classically is associated with normal female development, some cases of phenotypic males with this genetic constitution have been noted.

248. The answer is E (all). *(Williams, ed 5. pp 41-44.)* The gonadotropins (FSH and LH) are glycoproteins. In women, they stimulate the production of one or more primordial follicles and induce thecal cells in the ovary to produce estrogen. In a man who has hypopituitarism, the gonadotropins can cause production of spermatozoa and testosterone.

249. The answer is A (1, 2, 3). *(Williams, ed 5. p 46.)* Growth hormone and chorionic somatomammotropin are polypeptide hormones composed of 191 amino-acid subunits, of which 161 are identical (the other 30 are closely related and vary by only a simple base change in the DNA template). Although the structure of human prolactin is not yet clearly established, it too is a polypeptide hormone of close to 200 subunits, many of which are in the same sequence as the other two hormones. Prolactin, growth hormone, and chorionic somatomammotropin all are able to induce hormonal changes directly in their target organs. Thyrotropin is a glycoprotein; its only physiologic action is stimulation of the thyroid gland to produce another hormone, thyroxine, which is the mediator of thyroid activity.

250. The answer is D (4). *(Williams, ed 5. p 47.)* Levodopa can cause prolactin secretion to decrease. This compound increases the concentration of dopamine in the hypothalamus and, as a result, probably stimulates production of prolactin-release inhibiting factor. Alpha-methyldopa (which inhibits synthesis of dopamine), phenothiazines, reserpine, and probably serotonin all cause prolactin secretion to increase.

251. The answer is A (1, 2, 3). *(Speroff, p 161.)* The clinical symptoms and increased free cortisol levels of the woman described in the question suggest Cushing's disease. Her elevated cortisol levels also could be due to certain metabolical effects of birth-control pills. It was once believed that the pill increased the transcortin level but not the free cortisol level; however, the free cortisol level may in fact increase because of displacement of free cortisol from transcortin by progesterone. The high levels of estrogen in women taking birth-control pills can hinder the liver's ability to metabolize cortisol, resulting in higher-than-normal cortisol levels. If the pill has any effect on pituitary production of ACTH, it is a suppressive one.

252. The answer is E (all). *(Speroff, pp 142-143.)* Short stature can be associated with adrenal hyperplasia, Cushing's disease, and exogenous cortisone therapy. These factors cause short stature by increasing cortisol levels and, as a result, stimulating epiphyseal closure. Individuals who have Turner's syndrome also are characterized by short stature, due to a lack of estrogen production. Hypothyroidism and hypopituitarism can cause short stature in affected girls.

253. The answer is A (1, 2, 3). *(Speroff, p 162.)* Progestational agents in oral contraceptives work by a negative feedback mechanism to inhibit the secretion of hypothalamic releasing factor and, as a result, prevent ovulation. They also cause decidualization and atrophy of the endometrium, hence making implantation impossible. In addition, cervical mucus, which at ovulation is thin and watery, is changed by the influence of progestational agents to a tenacious compound that severely limits sperm motility; and some evidence indicates that they may change ovum and sperm migration patterns within the reproductive system. Progestins do not prevent irregular bleeding. Estrogen in birth-control pills enhances the negative feedback of the progestins and stabilizes the endometrium to prevent irregular menses.

254. The answer is C (2, 4). *(Speroff, pp 102-103.)* In the lactating breast, engorgement and milk production begin on the third or fourth postpartum day. Until this time, only colostrum, which is composed of desquamated epithelium and transudate, is manufactured. Transient increases in prolactin levels, which occur after delivery, are initiated by suckling and are crucial to the production of milk; once milk production has begun, however, prolactin levels in lactating as well as nonlactating women return rapidly to low levels. Oxytocin has very little, if any, role in the production of milk. Its primary function in lactation is initiation of milk letdown, which is a neural reflex in which suckling stimulates the myoepithelium of the breast to cause milk to be ejected.

255. The answer is A (1, 2, 3). *(Speroff, pp 103-104.)* The normal sequence of events triggered by suckling is as follows: Through a central-nervous-system response, dopamine is decreased in the hypothalamus. Dopamine suppression decreases production of prolactin inhibitory factor (PIF), which normally travels through a portal system to the pituitary gland; because PIF production is decreased, production of prolactin by the pituitary is increased. Suckling also suppresses the production of luteinizing-hormone releasing factor and, as a result, acts as a mild contraceptive (the midcycle LH surge does not occur).

256. The answer is A (1, 2, 3). *(Speroff, p 85.)* Estrogen withdrawal bleeding, estrogen breakthrough bleeding, and progesterone breakthrough bleeding are mechanisms of dysfunctional uterine bleeding, which is defined as bleeding that does not occur according to a normal cycle. Progesterone withdrawal bleeding is that mechanism by which normal menstrual flow commences. A woman normally ovulates on day 14, and the corpus luteum begins producing progesterone. When progesterone production ceases about 14 days later, menstruation ensues.

257. The answer is B (1, 3). *(Speroff, p 78.)* Asherman's syndrome is intrauterine synechia that usually follows a too-vigorous postpartum curettage. Affected women continue to ovulate, although they do not have menstrual bleeding; their basic body temperatures, therefore, are biphasic and normal. The diagnosis of Asherman's syndrome is made by hysteroscopy or by hysterosalpingography. The etiology is not related to insertion of an intrauterine device (IUD); however, IUDs are utilized in treatment, because they separate the walls of the uterus after the adhesions are broken. After placement of the IUDs, affected women should begin taking high doses of estrogen for three weeks a month, allowing the endometrium to regenerate.

258-262. The answers are: 258-B, 259-A, 260-C, 261-A, 262-D. *(Speroff, pp 86-90.)* The five phases of the ovulatory cycle describe the normal generation and degeneration of the endometrium without fertilization. The endometrium, including the stroma and especially the glands, undergoes active mitosis. This proliferative phase includes growth by mitotic division as well as by expansion of the stromal ground substance ("reinflation"). Stimulated by estrogen, the endometrium grows to a predetermined height, at which time the production of progesterone restrains the extent of the growth. Although endometrial height does not increase, growth of glands and vessels continues within the endometrium. The endometrium is now in the secretory phase. Implantation is made possible when the endometrium divides into three distinct layers: the basalis, the stratum spongiosum, and the stratum compacta. If no implantation occurs, the phase of endometrial breakdown occurs. This phase is characterized by vasoconstriction and vasodilatation of the spiral arterioles, causing hemorrhage into the stroma and necrosis. The tissue composing the stratum spongiosum and the stratum compacta is then shed from the endometrial lining and menstrual flow commences. The menstrual endometrium typically is shallow and dense, consisting mainly of basalis tissue and some spongiotic residues. This phase bridges the breakdown and proliferative phases.

263-268. The answers are: 263-C, 264-D, 265-B, 266-A, 267-A, 268-C. *(Speroff, pp 137-141. Williams, ed 5. pp 395-398, 808-813.)* True sexual precocity in girls is characterized by elevated gonadotropin levels and a normal ovulatory pattern. It represents premature activation of a normally operating hypothalamus-pituitary relationship. Although it usually is idiopathic, true sexual precocity can arise from cerebral causes as well as from hypothyroidism, polyostotic fibrous dysplasia, neurofibromatosis, and other disorders.

In girls who have precocious pseudopuberty, the endocrine glands, usually under neoplastic influences, produce elevated amounts of estrogens (isosexual precocious pseudopuberty) or androgens (heterosexual precocious pseudopuberty). Ovarian tumors appear to be the most common cause of isosexual precocious pseudopuberty; and some ovarian tumors, including dysgerminomas and choriocarcinomas, can produce so much gonadotropin that pregnancy tests are positive.

Incomplete sexual precocity, which usually is idiopathic, is characterized by only partial sexual maturity, such as premature thelarche, premature pubarche, or premature adrenarche. Incomplete sexual precocity can be accompanied by abnormal central-nervous-system function (e.g., mental deficiency).

In gonadotropin-producing tumors high levels of gonadotropins, such as FSH, are produced with subsequent production of estrogen. Examples of these tumors are hepatoma, chorioepithelioma, and presacral tumors.

269-273. The answers are: 269-B, 270-C, 271-E, 272-E, 273-D. *(Speroff, pp 152-158, 214-216.)* Ethinyl estradiol and mestranol are the two active synthetic estrogens used in birth-control pills (mestranol is employed more commonly than ethinyl estradiol). An ethinyl group at the 17 position makes these estrogens orally active.

By removing the 19 carbon from testosterone, a nontestosterone, orally active progestational agent (a 19-nortestosterone) is obtained. Norethindrone is the most commonly used progestational agent of this type in birth-control pills.

Medroxyprogesterone acetate (Provera), along with chlormadinone, has been noted to produce benign breast tumors in beagle puppies; when estrogens were administered at the same time, however, this effect could not be reproduced.

Clomiphene is a nonsteroidal antiestrogenic agent. By inhibiting hypothalamic regulation of estrogen production, causing estrogen levels to increase, clomiphene can promote ovulation in certain groups of anovulatory women.

274-277. The answers are: 274-C, 275-B, 276-E, 277-D. *(Speroff, pp 2-3.)* Cholesterol and all its steroid derivatives share the same basic molecular structure: a hydrogenated cyclopentophenanthrene-ring system, which is shown below.

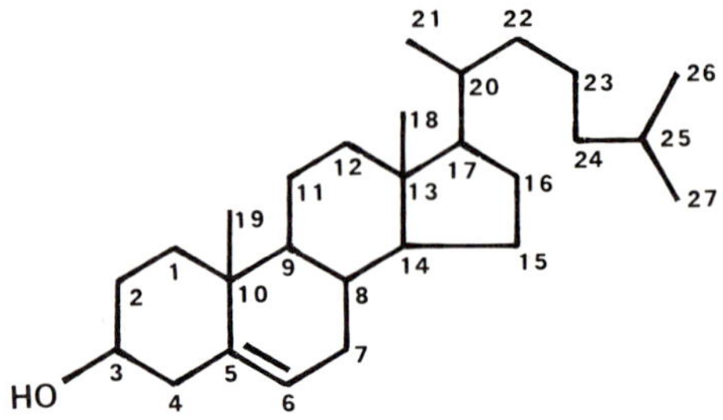

The number of carbon atoms, as well as the variations in size and position of side groups of the ring system, differentiate one steroid from another. For example, progestins and corticoids are 21-carbon compounds, and all estrogens are 18-carbon compounds.

278-282. The answers are: 278-A, 279-C, 280-B, 281-D, 282-D. *(Williams, ed 5. pp 276, 325, 330-332.)* Testosterone reaching a target organ, such as the prostate gland, is converted to dihydrotestosterone by 5α-reductase, an enzyme in the cell wall or cell membrane. Adenylcyclase, which is an intracellular enzyme activated by the presence of LH, catalyzes the formation of cyclic AMP, which then activates other intracellular enzyme reactions. The enzyme 17β-hydroxylase is found primarily in the testis but also in the adrenal gland; it converts androstenedione to testosterone by hydroxylating the 17 position.

The conversion of cholesterol into steroid hormones begins with hydroxylation at the 20 position followed by cleavage of the six-carbon side chain (carbons 22 to 27); both reactions, which result in production of pregnenolone, are catalyzed by 20-hydroxylase (also known as cholesterol desmolase). Congenital deficiencies of this enzyme can cause the adrenal glands to fill with cholesterol and become greatly enlarged; affected infants, some of whom may be phenotypic females but genotypic males, have a poor prognosis.

283-286. The answers are: 283-C, 284-D, 285-B, 286-A. *(Speroff, pp 92-93.)* The four women described represent the four different patterns of menstrual bleeding. The first woman is not ovulating, and because she is producing estrogen (in varying amounts) she continues to stimulate her endometrium; the endometrium grows to a point where it sloughs. This woman's bleeding thus is called estrogen breakthrough bleeding.

The second woman has estrogen withdrawal bleeding. She is producing very little estrogen or progesterone. Exogenous estrogen stimulates her endometrium to grow, but as soon as this stimulus is taken away the endometrium no longer has nutritive support and therefore is sloughed.

The third woman, who demonstrates progesterone withdrawal bleeding, represents a normally ovulating woman. At the end of 14 days, the corpus luteum stops producing progesterone and the endometrium loses its structural support and therefore is sloughed.

The fourth woman is taking birth-control pills and has a high progesterone-to-estrogen ratio. If the amount of progesterone is not high enough to support the endometrium in the early phases, and if structural support is poor, the endometrium will break down and the woman will have progesterone breakthrough bleeding.

287-291. The answers are: 287-C, 288-A, 289-C, 290-D, 291-B. *(Speroff, pp 42-43. Williams, ed 5. pp 234-236, 247-248, 328, 394.)* Under the influence of LH, testosterone is secreted by Leydig cells in the testis. Arrhenoblastomas, the most common androgen-secreting tumors of the ovary, produce and secrete testosterone; secretion of very small amounts of testosterone by this tumor can lead to virilization.

Steroid production in the ovary is by two pathways. Cells of the theca interna produce estrogen by a pathway in which pregnenolone is a key precursor. Granulosa cells, on the other hand, manufacture estrogen from progesterone.

Cortisol is a steroid produced by the adrenal cortex. Measurement of cortisol and some related steroids can be accomplished colorimetrically by reaction with phenylhydrazine in sulfuric acid, the so-called Porter-Silber reaction.

Obstetrics
General Considerations

Donald R. Coustan

Barney B. Silverman

DIRECTIONS: Each question below contains five suggested answers. Choose the **one best** response to each question.

292. At 12 weeks gestation, amniotic fluid volume is approximately

(A) 5 ml
(B) 20 ml
(C) 50 ml
(D) 100 ml
(E) 200 ml

293. At 13 weeks gestation, fetal weight is approximately

(A) 0.3 g
(B) 1 g
(C) 10 g
(D) 30 g
(E) 100 g

294. The normal umbilical cord contains which of the following systems of blood vessels?

(A) One artery and one vein
(B) One artery and two veins
(C) Two arteries and one vein
(D) Two arteries and two veins
(E) None of the above

295. During pregnancy a woman needs additional iron to satisfy the demands of the fetus, the placenta, and her own increasing hemoglobin mass. The total antepartum iron need is approximately

(A) 100 mg
(B) 250 mg
(C) 800 mg
(D) 1,200 mg
(E) 2,000 mg

Questions 296-298

The sketch shown below details the major landmarks of the fetal skull as it presents in the maternal pelvis. The perspective is that of the obstetrician facing the perineum.

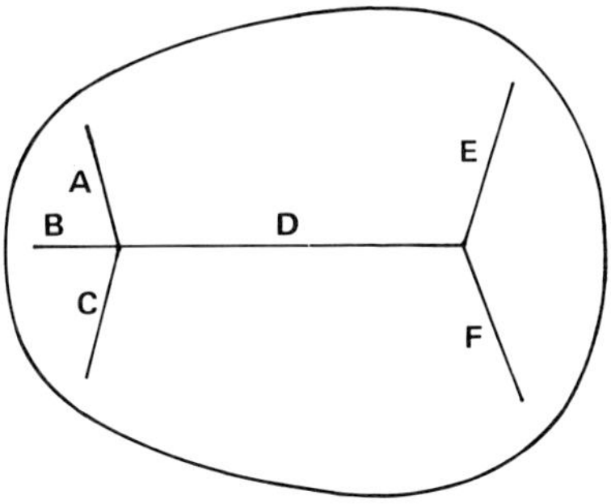

296. The position of the fetal vertex is

(A) left occiput anterior
(B) left sacrum transverse
(C) left occiput transverse
(D) right occiput transverse
(E) mentum posterior

297. The lambdoid sutures are

(A) **A** and **C**
(B) **A**, **C**, and **D**
(C) **B** and **D**
(D) **E** and **F**
(E) none of the above

298. The intersection of **D**, **E**, and **F** forms the

(A) caput succedaneum
(B) parietal prominence
(C) biparietal plane
(D) anterior fontanelle
(E) posterior fontanelle

Questions 299-301

A 24-year-old primigravid woman (28 weeks) develops spider angiomata, palmar erythema, and diffuse pruritus. You obtain a set of liver function tests, which reveal the following serum levels: alkaline phosphatase, 190 IU/l (normal: 21-91); glutamic oxaloacetic transaminase, 38 IU/l (normal: 6-18); total bilirubin, 1.8 mg/100 ml (normal: 0.3-1.0); direct bilirubin, 1.0 mg/100 ml (normal: 0.1-0.3).

299. Of the following diagnoses, which is the most likely for this woman?

(A) Cirrhosis
(B) Infectious hepatitis
(C) Cholestasis
(D) Acute pancreatitis
(E) Cholecystitis

300. The most appropriate treatment would be

(A) observation
(B) bed rest and high-protein diet
(C) oral corticosteroids
(D) low-fat diet
(E) oral cholestyramine

301. After delivery, the woman should be advised to

(A) avoid further pregnancies
(B) avoid high-fat foods
(C) avoid oral contraceptives
(D) have a cholecystectomy
(E) none of the above

302. The graph below depicts a labor curve for a woman, gravida 2, para 1, with intact membranes. This labor curve is compatible with which of the following conditions?

(A) Normal labor
(B) Protracted latent phase
(C) Protracted active phase
(D) Primary dysfunction
(E) Hypertonic dysfunction

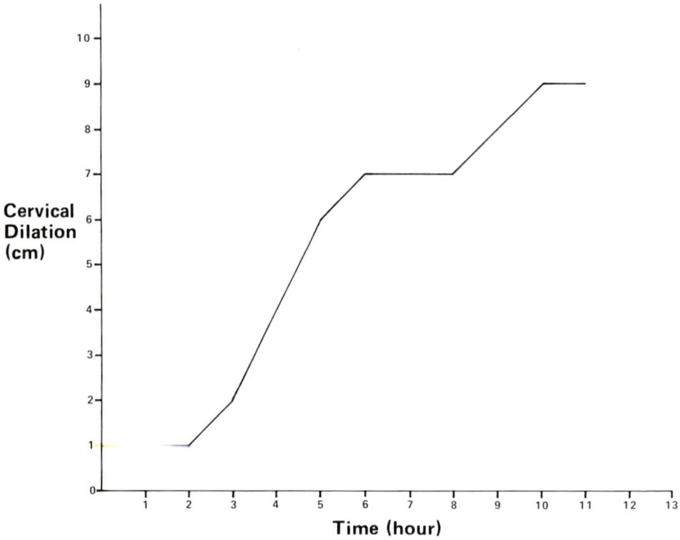

303. The cardinal movements of labor occur in which of the following sequences?

(A) Flexion, descent, internal rotation, external rotation, extension
(B) Flexion, descent, external rotation, internal rotation, extension
(C) Flexion, internal rotation, descent, extension, external rotation
(D) Descent, flexion, internal rotation, extension, external rotation
(E) Descent, flexion, external rotation, extension, internal rotation

304. Premature labor can be inhibited by the administration of all of the following agents EXCEPT

(A) betamethasone acetate
(B) ethanol
(C) β-adrenergic stimulators
(D) prostaglandin synthetase inhibitors
(E) 17-hydroxyprogesterone caproate

305. Which of the following statements about the third stage of labor is true?

(A) It is defined as the hour immediately following the delivery of the placenta
(B) The earliest clinical sign is that the uterus has become globular and firm
(C) Forced placental expression before placental separation often is beneficial
(D) There is less blood loss than normal with the Duncan mechanism of placental expression
(E) There is less blood loss than normal with Schultze's mechanism of placental expression

Questions 306-307

A 24-year-old primigravid woman, who is intent on breast feeding, decides upon a home delivery. Immediately after the birth of a 4.1-kilogram (nine-pound) infant, the patient bleeds massively due to extensive vaginal and cervical lacerations. She is brought in shock to the nearest hospital. Nine units of blood are transfused over two hours, and the blood pressure returns to a reasonable level. A hemoglobin value the next day is 7.5 g/100 ml, and three units of packed red blood cells are given.

306. One possible late sequela to consider in this woman would be

(A) hemochromatosis
(B) Stein-Leventhal syndrome
(C) Sheehan's syndrome
(D) Simmonds' syndrome
(E) Cushing's syndrome

307. Development of this sequela could be evident as early as

(A) 6 hours postpartum
(B) 1 week postpartum
(C) 1 month postpartum
(D) 6 months postpartum
(E) 1 year postpartum

308. A multiparous woman is one who has completed

(A) two or more pregnancies, regardless of the length of gestation
(B) two or more pregnancies reaching the stage of viability
(C) two or more pregnancies resulting in delivery
(D) two or more pregnancies resulting in delivery of liveborn infants
(E) a single pregnancy resulting in a multiple birth

309. During the first postpartum week, the uterus loses

(A) 10 percent of its immediate postpartum weight
(B) 25 percent of its immediate postpartum weight
(C) 50 percent of its immediate postpartum weight
(D) 75 percent of its immediate postpartum weight
(E) 90 percent of its immediate postpartum weight

310. The most common cause of uterine rupture during pregnancy is

(A) external trauma
(B) previous cesarean section
(C) previous myomectomy
(D) transverse lie
(E) stimulation of labor with oxytocin

311. The incidence of hydramnios is increased in association with all of the following EXCEPT

(A) fetal renal agenesis
(B) fetal esophageal atresia
(C) fetal anencephalus
(D) maternal diabetes mellitus
(E) presence of monozygotic twins

312. The oxytocin challenge test is considered negative if

(A) at least three uterine contractions occur in a ten-minute interval and late deceleration of fetal heart rate is absent
(B) at least three uterine contractions occur in a ten-minute interval and late deceleration is inconsistent
(C) less than three uterine contractions occur in a ten-minute interval, regardless of whether late deceleration occurs
(D) the uterus contracts at least once every two minutes, regardless of whether late deceleration occurs
(E) no uterine contractions are noted

313. Which of the following statements about frank breech presentation is true?

(A) It is less common than complete breech presentation
(B) It is less common than incomplete breech presentation
(C) The lower extremities are flexed at the hips but extended at the knees
(D) The hips and one or both knees are flexed
(E) The feet often can be palpated beside the buttocks

314. A 25-year-old woman, gravida 1, para 0, who has a history of infertility, comes to your office at 20 weeks by dates. Her uterus in enlarged (24-weeks). She was treated in the past with a fertility drug, the name of which she does not know. You obtain an ultrasonogram, which is shown below. The most likely diagnosis is

(A) hydatidiform mole
(B) placenta previa
(C) anencephalic fetus
(D) twins
(E) normal single-fetus pregnancy

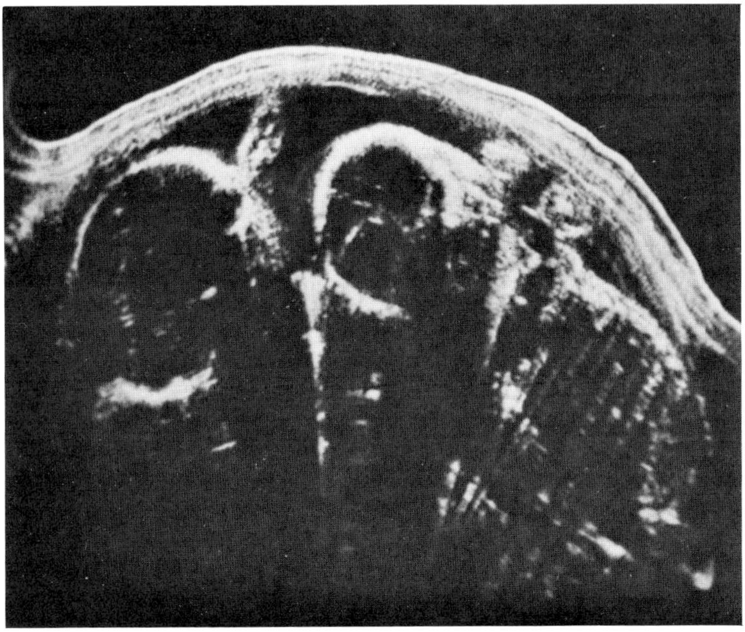

DIRECTIONS: Each question below contains four suggested answers of which **one** or **more** is correct. Choose the answer:

A	if	**1, 2, and 3**	are correct
B	if	**1 and 3**	are correct
C	if	**2 and 4**	are correct
D	if	**4**	is correct
E	if	**1, 2, 3, and 4**	are correct

315. Barton forceps can be described by which of the following statements?

(1) It is useful when the fetal head is in a transverse position in a platypelloid pelvis
(2) It is useful when traction and rotation are to be performed simultaneously
(3) Application of the blades can be adjusted by a sliding lock
(4) The posterior blade is hinged

316. Which of the following statements describing toxoplasmosis in a pregnant woman are true?

(1) It can be acquired by eating infected meat that is raw or uncooked
(2) It occurs in one in every 2,000 to 2,500 pregnancies
(3) Infection in early pregnancy may lead to abortion
(4) Transplacental infection of the fetus is highly unlikely

317. Obstetric analgesia and anesthesia can be described by which of the following statements?

(1) The most common cause of death due to anesthesia is pneumonitis from aspirated gastric material and juices
(2) Intravenous thiopental and other barbiturates are relatively ineffective in producing analgesia and can cause depression in the newborn infant
(3) Antacids given before general anesthesia can diminish the risk of serious pulmonary injury
(4) Naloxone, a narcotic antagonist, is effective only against respiratory depression induced by opioid narcotics

318. In a lower uterine segment cesarean section, the advantages of a transverse incision as compared to a vertical incision include

(1) less blood loss
(2) less likelihood of extending into the broad ligaments
(3) less likelihood of extending into the cervix and vagina
(4) more room for extraction of the fetus

319. Common findings in the "incompetent cervix" syndrome include

(1) painless dilatation of the cervix
(2) a history of cervical trauma
(3) spontaneous rupture of the membranes at midpregnancy
(4) recurrent pregnancy loss at 14 to 16 weeks gestation

320. Fetal presenting positions that are usually undeliverable include

(1) brow
(2) mentum anterior
(3) mentum posterior
(4) left sacrum posterior

321. Predisposing factors to face presentation include

(1) large fetus
(2) contracted pelvis
(3) pendulous abdomen
(4) anencephalic fetus

322. Premature separation of the placenta occurs more commonly than normal in association with which of the following conditions?

(1) Previous abruptio placentae
(2) Chronic hypertension
(3) Toxemia of pregnancy
(4) Delivery of twins

323. A 27-year-old woman, gravida 3, para 2, comes to the delivery floor at 37 weeks gestation by dates. She has had no prenatal care. She complains that, on bending down to pick up her two-year-old child, she experienced sudden, severe back pain. This pain now has persisted for two hours. Approximately 30 minutes ago she noted bright red blood coming from her vagina. By the time she arrives at the delivery floor, she is contracting strongly every three minutes; the uterus is quite firm even between contractions. By abdominal palpation the fetus is vertex with the head deeply engaged. Fetal heart rate is 130 beats per minute. The fundus is 38 cm above the symphysis. Blood for clotting is drawn, and a clot forms in four minutes. Clotting studies are sent. The best course of action would be

(1) rupture of membranes
(2) stimulation of labor with oxytocin solution
(3) attachment of internal scalp electrode and insertion of intrauterine catheter for monitoring
(4) immediate administration of heparin

324. Which of the following circumstances should alert an obstetrician to an increased likelihood of postpartum hemorrhage?

(1) Prolonged labor
(2) Rapid labor
(3) Oxytocin stimulation of labor
(4) Twin pregnancy

SUMMARY OF DIRECTIONS

A	B	C	D	E
1, 2, 3 only	1, 3 only	2, 4 only	4 only	All are correct

325. Signs of placental separation include which of the following?

(1) Lengthening of the umbilical cord
(2) Change in the shape of the uterus from globular to discoid
(3) Sudden gush of blood
(4) Strong uterine contractions

326. The human placenta produces which of the following hormones?

(1) Gonadotropin
(2) Somatomammotropin
(3) Progesterone
(4) Hydrocortisone

327. Positive signs of pregnancy include which of the following?

(1) Ultrasonographic visualization of the fetal head
(2) Detection of the funic souffle
(3) Perception of fetal movements by an experienced examiner
(4) Positive urine test for chorionic gonadotropin

328. A group of congenital anomalies known collectively as Potter's syndrome includes renal agenesis (or other renal anomalies) and pulmonary hypoplasia. Other anomalies associated with Potter's syndrome include

(1) hydrocephaly
(2) amnion nodosum
(3) cleft palate
(4) oligohydramnios

329. Hypertonic dysfunctional labor generally can be expected to

(1) cause little pain
(2) occur in the active phase of labor
(3) react favorably to oxytocin
(4) respond to sedation

330. Precipitate labor, which most often occurs in multiparous women, is associated with a greater-than-normal incidence of which of the following?

(1) Amniotic fluid embolism
(2) Fetal hypoxia
(3) Fetal cerebral trauma
(4) Cervical laceration

331. The amount of estriol in a maternal 24-hour urine sample may be decreased due to

(1) the administration of oral ampicillin
(2) the administration of oral corticosteroids
(3) maternal pyelonephritis
(4) placental sulfatase deficiency

332. Prerequisites for application of forceps include

(1) complete dilation of the cervix
(2) engagement
(3) ruptured membranes
(4) vertex or face presentation

333. An infant born at term has a heart rate greater than 100 per minute one minute after birth. Also at this time, respiration is judged to be slow and irregular, extremities are blue and show some flexion, and the cry is weak; the body (except for the extremities) is pink. Which of the following statements about this infant are true?

(1) The one-minute Apgar score is 6
(2) An infant having a higher one-minute Apgar score would be more severely depressed
(3) Mild to moderate respiratory depression is present
(4) Resuscitation should be started immediately

334. As a description of a woman's obstetric history, the digits 7-2-1-6 indicate that she

(1) has given birth to six term infants
(2) has had two premature deliveries
(3) has been pregnant seven times
(4) has had one abortion

335. Which of the following statements about monozygotic twinning are true?

(1) It tends to run in families
(2) It frequently is associated with pregnancies induced by clomiphene citrate
(3) It is more common than dizygotic twinning
(4) It occurs in approximately 1 pregnancy in 250

336. Substances that are normally found in higher concentrations in maternal blood than in fetal or umbilical cord blood include

(1) immunoglobulin G (IgG)
(2) immunoglobulin M (IgM)
(3) gamma chains of hemoglobin
(4) fibrinogen

337. Which of the following statements about bacteriuria in pregnant women are true?

(1) It characteristically is first noted early in pregnancy
(2) It greatly increases the risk of prematurity
(3) The prevalence of asymptomatic bacteriuria during pregnancy has been found to vary according to race, parity, and socioeconomic status
(4) One-half of women who have asymptomatic bacteriuria subsequently develop acute symptomatic bacteriuria during pregnancy

SUMMARY OF DIRECTIONS

A	B	C	D	E
1, 2, 3 only	1, 3 only	2, 4 only	4 only	All are correct

338. Infection of the genital tract after delivery of an infant (puerperal infection) can be described by which of the following statements?

(1) A temperature of 38°C (100.4°F) or higher on any two of the first ten postpartum days (excluding the first day) is considered the standard definition of puerperal morbidity
(2) Iatrogenic causes are significant sources of infection
(3) The most common pathogens involved are those that normally inhabit the bowel and lower genital tract
(4) Anaerobic infections are common and frequently are caused by *Bacteroides*, *Peptostreptococcus*, or *Clostridium*

339. Pregnant women who have diabetes mellitus are affected by which of the following conditions more often than nondiabetic women?

(1) Pre-eclampsia and eclampsia
(2) Infection
(3) Postpartum hemorrhage after vaginal delivery
(4) Hydramnios

340. Which of the following statements about the oxytocin challenge test are true?

(1) It determines the inducability of the uterus
(2) Its effects are measured by internal monitors
(3) It is considered positive if the uterus contracts once every two minutes
(4) It can serve as a fetal stress test

341. Vaginal delivery accompanied by which of the following conditions is likely to result in compromise of the infant?

(1) Prolapse of the umbilical cord
(2) Shoulder presentation
(3) Persistent brow presentation
(4) Persistent occiput posterior position

342. Common causes of immediate postpartum hemorrhage include which of the following?

(1) Uterine atony
(2) Retained placental fragments
(3) Vaginal lacerations
(4) Congenital uterine anomalies

343. Which of the following laboratory values can be expected to increase during pregnancy?

(1) Serum albumin
(2) Plasma fibrinogen
(3) Blood urea nitrogen
(4) Erythrocyte sedimentation rate

DIRECTIONS: The groups of questions below consist of lettered choices followed by several numbered items. For each numbered item select the **one** lettered choice with which it is **most** closely associated. Each lettered choice may be used once, more than once, or not at all.

Questions 344-348

For each description that follows, select the disorder with which it is most likely to be associated.

(A) Placental polyps
(B) Placenta previa
(C) Abruptio placentae
(D) Ectopic pregnancy
(E) Spontaneous abortion

344. Associated with the Arias-Stella phenomenon

345. Premature placental separation

346. Associated with maternal hypertension

347. May be due to defective vascularization of the decidua caused by inflammation or atrophy

348. Usually accompanied by thickened placental villi, hemorrhage into the decidua basalis, and evidence of necrosis in tissues near the bleeding

Questions 349-351

For each of the following clinical descriptions, select the procedure that would be most appropriate.

(A) External version
(B) Internal version
(C) Midforceps rotation
(D) Low transverse cesarean section
(E) Classical cesarean section

349. A 24-year-old primigravid woman, at term, has been in labor for 16 hours and has been 9 cm dilated for 3 hours. The fetal vertex is in the right occiput posterior position, at +1 station, and molded. There have been mild late decelerations for the last 30 minutes. Twenty minutes ago, the fetal scalp pH was 7.27; it is now 7.20

350. A 24-year-old woman, gravida 3, para 2, is at 40 weeks gestation. The fetus is in the transverse lie presentation

351. You have just delivered a 2.5-kilogram (5.5-pound) baby at 39 weeks gestation. Because the uterus still feels large, you do a vaginal examination. A second set of membranes is bulging through a fully dilated cervix, and you feel a small part presenting in the sac. A fetal heart is auscultated at 60 beats per minute

Questions 352-354

For each of the descriptions below, select the pelvic type with which it is most likely to be associated.

(A) Anthropoid
(B) Android
(C) Gynecoid
(D) Platypelloid
(E) None of the above

352. Examination of the pelvis reveals prominent ischial spines, a narrow subpubic arch, a narrow high-arched sacrosciatic notch, a straight sacrum, and a shortened posterior sagittal diameter

353. Examination of the pelvis reveals a wide subpubic arch, a curved sacrum, and a shortened anteroposterior diameter

354. Examination of the pelvis reveals a lengthened anteroposterior diameter, a large sacrosciatic notch, prominent ischial spines, and a straight, posteriorly inclined sacrum

Questions 355-358

For each of the following substances, choose the mechanism of transplacental transport most likely to be employed.

(A) Simple diffusion
(B) Facilitated diffusion
(C) Active transport
(D) Pinocytosis
(E) None of the above

355. Carbon dioxide

356. Iron

357. Oxygen

358. Glucose

Questions 359-363

Whether it is safe to receive immunizations during pregnancy is a matter of concern and controversy; and the question has prompted the American College of Obstetricians and Gynecologists to offer specific recommendations for the use of immunization therapy for pregnant women. For each disease vaccine that follows, select the recommendation with which it is most likely to be associated.

(A) Recommended if the underlying disease is serious
(B) Recommended after exposure or before travel to endemic areas
(C) Not routinely recommended but mandatory during an epidemic
(D) Contraindicated unless exposure to the disease is unavoidable
(E) Contraindicated

359. Poliomyelitis

360. Mumps

361. Influenza

362. Rubella

363. Hepatitis-A

Questions 364-366

For each clinical situation that follows, select the most likely placental disorder.

(A) Vasa praevia
(B) Placenta succenturiata
(C) Placenta circumvallata
(D) Placenta membranacea
(E) Placenta accreta

364. A 24-year-old woman, gravida 2, para 1, goes into premature labor at 33 weeks after an apparently normal antepartum course

365. An apparently normal pregnancy culminates in the spontaneous delivery of a 3.2-kilogram (seven-pound) infant with Apgars 9/9. The placenta delivers spontaneously, but afterwards an unusual amount of uterine bleeding occurs

366. After the low forceps delivery of a 1.8-kilogram (four-pound) infant to a 27-year-old woman, gravida 4, para 3 (whose second baby was born by cesarean section due to fetal distress but whose third baby delivered vaginally), the placenta does not deliver spontaneously. After 20 minutes the obstetrician attempts a manual removal but is unable to identify a plane of cleavage

Questions 367-369

For each description below, choose the appropriate type of obstetric forceps.

(A) Simpson's forceps
(B) Kielland's forceps
(C) Barton forceps
(D) Chamberlen forceps
(E) Tarnier's forceps

367. These forceps were designed for the occiput transverse position in a flat pelvis

368. These forceps were designed for rotation; their pelvic curve is almost nonexistent

369. These forceps are useful for an elective low forceps delivery

Obstetrics
General Considerations

Answers

292. The answer is C. *(Pritchard, ed 15. p 166.)* At 12 weeks gestation, amniotic fluid volume is approximately 50 ml, rapidly increasing to about 200 ml by 16 weeks. For this reason, pregnancy termination by intra-amniotic instillation of saline or prostaglandin solutions is extremely difficult at 12 weeks but becomes relatively simple beyond 16 weeks. Because termination by suction abortion is dangerous beyond 12 weeks, the month between 12 and 16 weeks is a time when no method is safe.

293. The answer is D. *(Pritchard, ed 15. p 164.)* At 13 weeks gestation, the end of the first trimester, the developing fetus weighs approximately 30 g and is approximately 8 cm in length. That most major body structures have formed by this time is useful information in evaluating the duration of pregnancy in a spontaneous abortion. Most teratogenic influences, it should be noted, occur prior to this time.

294. The answer is C. *(Pritchard, ed 15. p 473.)* The normal umbilical cord contains two arteries and one vein. The absence of one umbilical artery is found in less than 1 percent of all babies. Although the significance of a missing umbilical artery is somewhat controversial, absence of the artery may indicate that other congenital anomalies also are present. Therefore, the obstetrician must verify the number of umbilical vessels and notify the pediatrician of any abnormality.

295. The answer is C. *(Pritchard, ed 15. pp 182-183.)* The fetus and placenta contain approximately 300 mg of elemental iron at birth. In addition, the maternal increase in hemoglobin mass accounts for about 500 mg of elemental iron. Thus, the total antepartum iron requirement is 800 mg. Most of this iron is needed during the second half of pregnancy, at an approximate rate of 5.7 mg daily during the last 140 days. However, because about 1 mg of iron is excreted daily, the total daily iron need is almost 7 mg during the second half of pregnancy. Most women of childbearing age cannot mobilize this much iron, and supplemental iron must be given to prevent iron deficiency. The usual iron supplement, ferrous sulfate, contains 20 percent elemental iron. Thus, a 325 mg tablet contains about 65 mg of elemental iron, of which 10 to 20 percent will be absorbed. Most prenatal vitamins contain 60 or 65 mg of iron, and these should be adequate for a healthy pregnant woman. If iron stores have been depleted by poor dietary habits, recent childbirth, or other causes, however, additional iron supplementation may be necessary.

296-298. The answers are: 296-C, 297-D, 298-E. *(Pritchard, ed 15. pp 148, 235-236.)* A good knowledge of the major landmarks of the fetal skull is essential for anyone performing deliveries. The position of the fetal vertex in the accompanying sketch is left occiput transverse. The lambdoid sutures (**E** and **F**) meet the sagittal suture (**D**) to form the posterior fontanelle. The occiput is just posterior to the posterior fontanelle. The posterior, or Y-shaped, fontanelle is the reference point for vertex presentations. The side of the maternal pelvis to which it is closest defines the position. The head is oriented in a transverse (or horizontal) manner, with the occiput nearest the maternal left side; thus, this is left occiput transverse. The anterior, or diamond-shaped, fontanelle, is made up of the intersection of the sagittal, frontal (**B**), and the two coronal (**A** and **C**) sutures. Extreme molding of the fetal head may make identification of these landmarks extremely difficult. Other clues to the position of the head include abdominal palpation of the back and small parts and, more important, palpation of an ear. If an ear can be felt and the relationship between the locations of the pinna and the auditory canal can be ascertained, the position of the vertex can be deduced.

299-301. The answers are: 299-C, 300-E, 301-C. *(Pritchard, ed 15. pp 195-196, 632-633.)* The most likely diagnosis for the woman described is cholestatic jaundice of pregnancy (cholestasis). Spider angiomata and palmar erythema are normal occurrences in pregnant women and do not imply hepatic disease. Generalized pruritus in pregnancy, however, may be caused by cholestasis. In this disorder, bilirubin may or may not be elevated; and elevation, if present, is usually only to a mild degree. Although serum alkaline phosphatase levels may double during normal pregnancy, it is usually even higher in cholestasis of pregnancy. If placental (heat-stable) alkaline phosphatase can be distinguished from the hepatic isozyme, then hepatic alkaline phosphatase will show an increase in patients with cholestasis. Levels of serum glutamic-oxaloacetic transaminase may be mildly elevated.

The appropriate treatment for this condition, if the itching is intractable, is oral cholestyramine, an exchange resin that ties up bile salts in the gastrointestinal tract and presumably reduces their levels in the periphery. Although its safety in pregnancy is not unequivocally established, oral cholestyramine is commonly used for this condition when treatment is necessary.

Cholestasis tends to recur in subsequent pregnancies and to accompany use of oral contraceptives. If the patient is willing to go through another pregnancy with the symptoms described, it is not contraindicated; however, oral contraceptives are probably a poor choice for family planning in these patients. In the case described, there is no reason to suspect pancreatitis; cirrhosis does not tend to be exacerbated by pregnancy; the enzyme values do not support hepatitis; and the patient does not show symptoms of cholecystitis.

302. The answer is C. *(Pritchard, ed 15. p 658.)* The labor described by the curve is characteristic of a protracted active phase. That the woman has entered the active phase is evident by the rate of dilatation (from 2 cm to 7 cm) over the space of three hours. The normal active phase progresses at a rate of at least 1.5 cm/hr in a multiparous woman and 1.2 cm/hr in a nulliparous woman. After 7 cm dilatation is reached in this patient, however, progress slows down to 2 cm over the next four hours, or 0.5 cm/hr, and the active phase is said to be protracted. Another name for this condition is secondary arrest of labor. (Primary arrest of labor is arrest of progress before the active phase has begun.) If this woman's contractions are adequate by intrauterine monitoring and further progress does not occur, most obstetricians would perform a cesarean section. If hypotonic dysfunction were causing the protracted labor, some obstetricians would stimulate contractions with intravenous oxytocin.

303. The answer is D. *(Pritchard, ed 15. pp 315-317.)* Although the cardinal movements of labor do not necessarily follow one after another, they may be sequenced to aid in understanding labor's underlying mechanisms. The head generally enters the pelvis as an occiput transverse presentation, due to the usual configuration of the inlet. As it **descends** into the pelvis, **flexion** occurs. As the head passes the midplane, the musculature of the pelvic floor causes **internal rotation**, or movement from occiput transverse to occiput anterior (or posterior). As the occiput passes under the symphysis and comes in contact with the perineum, **extension** occurs, allowing delivery of the head. As the shoulders pass into the pelvis, they align in the anteroposterior plane, causing the head to go back to the occiput transverse position, a process called **external rotation.**

304. The answer is A. *(Pritchard, ed 15. pp 792-794.)* Ethanol, certain beta-adrenergic stimulators (e.g., salbutamol), agents that block prostaglandin synthesis (e.g., indomethacin), and progestational agents (e.g., 17-hydroxyprogesterone caproate) all have been used with some success to inhibit premature labor. Betamethasone acetate, when administered to women whose membranes have ruptured earlier than the 32nd week of gestation and who are given labor-inhibiting medications, significantly reduces the incidence of respiratory distress syndrome in the infants subsequently delivered.

305. The answer is B. *(Pritchard, ed 15. pp 313, 340-342.)* The third stage of labor is the period between delivery of the infant and separation of the placenta. The characteristic signs of placental separation usually occur within five minutes of delivery; in order of appearance, these signs include firming of a globular uterus, a gush of blood, uterine ascent in the abdomen, and lengthening of the umbilical cord. Forced expression of the placenta before it has separated can be dangerous, because it can cause inversion of the uterus. Schultze's mechanism and the Duncan mechanism refer to variations of placental expulsion; neither is associated with decreased blood loss.

306-307. The answers are: 306-C, 307-B. *(Pritchard, ed 15. p 746.)* A disadvantage of home delivery is the lack of facilities to control postpartum hemorrhage. The woman described in the question delivered a large baby, suffered multiple soft-tissue injuries, and went into shock, needing nine units of blood by the time she reached the hospital. Sheehan's syndrome seems a likely possibility in this woman. This syndrome of anterior pituitary necrosis related to obstetrical hemorrhage can be diagnosed by one week postpartum, as lactation fails to commence normally. Although many modern women choose hormonal therapy in order to prevent lactation, the patient discussed was intent on breast feeding and so would not have received suppressant. She therefore could have been expected to begin lactation at the usual time. Other symptoms of Sheehan's syndrome include amenorrhea, atrophy of the breasts, and loss of thyroid and adrenal function.

The other presented choices for late sequelae are rather far-fetched. Hemochromatosis would not be expected to occur in this healthy young woman, especially since she did not receive prolonged transfusions. Cushing's, Simmonds', and Stein-Leventhal syndromes are not known to be related to postpartum hemorrhage.

It is important to note that home delivery is **not** a predisposing factor to postpartum hemorrhage.

308. The answer is B. *(Pritchard, ed 15. p 246.)* Parity is determined by the number of pregnancies that have reached viability (i.e., beyond the stage of abortion) and not by the number of deliveries. Parity is not increased by a multiple birth or decreased by a stillbirth.

309. The answer is C. *(Pritchard, ed 15. pp 374-376.)* At the time of delivery, the uterus weighs approximately 1,000 grams. By 1 week postpartum the weight is down to 500 grams; by 4 to 6 weeks postpartum it is back to its normal weight, less than 100 grams. Most of the weight loss is due to diminution in cell size rather than cell number. Clinically, it is important to keep these facts in mind when examining patients after delivery. If the uterus is still enlarged at the time of the postpartum checkup (usually six weeks), a pathologic process, such as subinvolution of the placental site or retained secundines, must be suspected.

310. The answer is B. *(Pritchard, ed 15. pp 729-730.)* More than any other factor, delivery by cesarean section in an earlier pregnancy predisposes a woman to uterine rupture in subsequent pregnancies. Oxytocin stimulation of labor also is associated with rupture of the uterus and, in fact, may be the second most common cause. Other factors associated less frequently with uterine rupture include previous myomectomy, external trauma (such as an accident or bullet wound), breech delivery, and congenital or acquired defects of the uterus.

311. The answer is A. *(Pritchard, ed 15. p 476.)* Hydramnios has been defined as the presence of more than 2,000 ml of amniotic fluid (normally, a peak amniotic fluid volume of about 1 liter is reached by 36 weeks gestation). Conditions that are associated with an increased incidence of hydramnios include twin pregnancies, particularly of monozygotic twins, maternal diabetes mellitus, and erythroblastosis fetalis; developmental abnormalities in the fetus, especially of the gastrointestinal tract and central nervous system, also are accompanied commonly by the presence of hydramnios. Reduced amniotic fluid volume (oligohydramnios) has been associated with renal agenesis.

312. The answer is A. *(Pritchard, ed 15. pp 281-282.)* The oxytocin challenge test is negative if the uterus contracts at least three times in a ten-minute interval, if each contraction lasts 40 seconds or longer, and if the contractions are not accompanied by a late deceleration of the fetal heart rate. A test result is considered suspicious if late deceleration is uneven and unsustained in spite of continuing uterine contraction. In the presence of hyperstimulation of the uterus, judged either by the contraction frequency (more than one every two minutes) or length (longer than 90 seconds), late deceleration of the fetal heart rate may not signify uteroplacental disease.

313. The answer is C. *(Pritchard, ed 15. p 666.)* The position of the lower extremities relative to the buttocks helps determine the descriptive presentation of the breech. Frank breech presentation is characterized by flexion of the lower extremities at the hips and extension at the knees. With a complete breech presentation, the hips and one or both knees are flexed; often, feet can be felt beside the buttocks. In incomplete breech presentation, the hips are not flexed and at least one foot or knee lies below the breech. Radiographic diagnosis of frank breech presentation is more common than of either complete or incomplete breech.

314. The answer is D. *(Pritchard, ed 15. pp 529-550.)* The ultrasonogram presented in the question clearly shows twins. The diagnosis can be made by noting the two heads (the circular densities). A hydatidiform mole would show no evidence of fetal parts or cranium. The presence of a spherical cranium rules out anencephaly. Because the placenta is anterior and superior, placenta previa is not present. Ultrasound has been very helpful in the diagnosis, early in gestation, of twins.

315. The answer is B (1, 3). *(Pritchard, ed 15. p 880.)* A special feature of Barton forceps is the hinged anterior blade. This type of forceps is useful when the fetal head is in a transverse position in a platypelloid pelvis; it should not be used, however, to perform simultaneous traction and rotation. Application of the forceps is by moving the hinged blade about the occiput or face; adjustment is made by a sliding lock.

316. The answer is B (1, 3). *(Pritchard, ed 15. p 640.)* Toxoplasmosis, a protozoal infection caused by *Toxoplasma gondii*, can result from ingestion of raw or undercooked meat infected by the organism or from contact with infected cat feces. Its incidence in pregnant women is estimated to be one in every 150 to 700 pregnancies. Infection early in pregnancy may cause abortion; later in pregnancy, however, the fetus may become infected. A small number of infected infants develop involvement of the central nervous system or the eye; most infants who have the disease, however, escape serious clinical problems.

317. The answer is E (all). *(Pritchard, ed 15. pp 354-358.)* In obstetrics, death from anesthesia most commonly results from pneumonitis caused by the inhalation of gastric acid. Administration of antacids before general anesthesia can lessen gastric acidity and therefore reduce the risk of serious pulmonary injury. The use of intravenous thiopental or other barbiturates, which are rather ineffective analgesics, can cause significant respiratory depression in the newborn. Narcotic antagonists, such as naloxone, levallorphan, and nalorphine, are effective only in reducing respiratory depression caused by opioid narcotics.

318. The answer is B (1, 3). *(Pritchard, ed 15. p 906.)* In a lower uterine segment cesarean section, a transverse incision results in less blood loss, because it goes through the thinned-out lower uterine segment and does not involve much of the myometrium, site of the large blood vessels. (However, if the placenta is implanted over the anterior lower uterine segment, blood loss can be significant.) The transverse incision also is less likely to extend into the cervix and vagina, because its direction of extension is usually horizontal. A transverse incision is more likely than a vertical incision to extend into the broad ligaments. If this happens, catastrophic hemorrhage can result. A vertical incision actually allows more room for extraction of the fetus, because it can extend upward toward the fundus. Many obstetricians prefer the vertical incision in situations where extra room is needed, as in a breech, for example.

319. The answer is A (1, 2, 3). *(Pritchard, ed 15. pp 493-495.)* When an incompetent cervix is suspected, weekly cervical examinations beginning at 16 to 18 weeks gestation can reveal evidence of cervical dilatation or effacement in time to perform corrective surgery. The most commonly used techniques are the Shirodkar cervical suture (circlage), in which the pursestring suture is buried under the vaginal mucosa and the bladder pushed back for higher placement of the stitch, and the McDonald cervical suture, a simple pursestring suture most widely used when the cervix is well effaced. Once the diagnosis has been made, a circlage procedure may be performed prophylactically in subsequent pregnancies, prior to any change in the cervix. This is best done at 14 to 16 weeks, well past the time when spontaneous abortion is common. Because it is not until 16 to 18 weeks that the fetus begins to occupy the lower uterine segment, it would be unlikely that incompetent cervix would be the cause of recurrent pregnancy loss at 14 to 16 weeks.

320. The answer is B (1, 3). *(Pritchard, ed 15. pp 676-681.)* In brow presentation, the fetal head is midway between flexion and extension. Except with an extremely small baby, engagement cannot occur unless flexion to vertex or extension to face presentation supervenes. In face presentation, delivery is by flexion rather than extension as in vertex presentations. Only the mentum anterior is capable of flexing under the pubic symphysis. The mentum posterior position does not allow flexion, because the neck is too short to go around the sacrum. The left sacrum posterior position is a variation of breech presentation. Although many present-day obstetricians would rarely deliver a breech vaginally, the breech presentation is by no means undeliverable.

321. The answer is E (all). *(Pritchard, ed 15. pp 676-677.)* Face presentations occur in approximately 0.2 percent of deliveries. A large or anencephalic fetus, contracted pelvis, and pendulous abdomen all make extension of the head more likely. In addition, tumors of the anterior neck or multiple coils of umbilical cord around the neck may predispose to face presentation. Cesarean section commonly is made necessary by face presentation; it may be avoided in many cases, however, if the decision is put off until the second stage of labor, when flexion or rotation to the mentum anterior position may occur.

322. The answer is E (all). *(Pritchard, ed 15. pp 407-416.)* Premature separation of the placenta (abruptio placentae) occurs in approximately 1 percent of all deliveries. Previous abruptio placentae, chronic hypertension, and toxemia of pregnancy all predispose to premature separation of the placenta. The placenta also is more likely than normal to separate between the birth of a first and second twin. Clinically, the severity of abruption ranges from a minimal amount of vaginal bleeding and rapid labor to massive hemorrhage, shock, consumptive coagulopathy, and fetal death. Clinical signs of abruption include an irritable, tender uterus, an enlarging uterus, hypertonic labor, and abdominal pain. Vaginal bleeding may or may not be present; in fact, some of the most severe abruptions with coagulopathies occur with "concealed hemorrhage," in which the retroplacental clot is contained within the uterus and has no egress to the vagina.

323. The answer is B (1, 3). *(Pritchard, ed 15. pp 406-416.)* The patient described presents with a classic history for abruption, the sudden onset of abdominal pain accompanied by bleeding. Physical examination, which reveals a firm, tender uterus with frequent contractions, confirms the diagnosis. The fact that a clot forms within four minutes suggests that coagulopathy is not present. Cesarean section may be necessary in the case of a severe abruption, but only when fetal distress is evident or delivery is unlikely to be accomplished vaginally. Internal monitoring equipment should provide an early warning that the fetus is compromised. The internal uterine catheter provides pressure recordings, which are important if use of oxytocin is necessary. Generally, however, patients with abruptio placentae are contracting vigorously and do not need oxytocin stimulation.

324. The answer is E (all). *(Pritchard, ed 15. p 473.)* Prolonged or rapid labor, oxytocin stimulation of labor, and twin pregnancy all predipose to uterine atony and, thus, to postpartum hemorrhage. A uterus that has required oxytocin in order to provide adequate labor is likely to need large amounts of oxytocin afterwards in order to stay contracted. A uterus that has stretched to accommodate twin gestations is likely to be atonic after it is emptied. No explanation is given for the clinical finding that a uterus that has been hypertonic and yielded a rapid labor is predisposed to atony.

325. The answer is B (1, 3). *(Pritchard, ed 15. p 340.)* The usual signs of placental separation include lengthening of the umbilical cord, a sudden gush of blood, a change in the shape of the uterus from discoid to globular, and the rising up of the uterus in the abdomen. Attempts to deliver the placenta before separation may cause serious problems, such as inversion of the uterus or avulsion of the cord. One useful way to avoid inverting the uterus is to wait until the placenta has separated and is in the lower uterine segment and then to perform the Brandt (or Brandt-Andrews) maneuver, pressing upward on the fundus from the suprapubic region while gently exerting cord traction.

326. The answer is A (1, 2, 3). *(Pritchard, ed 15. pp 123-135.)* The polypeptide hormones, human chorionic gonadotropin and human chorionic somatomammotropin (HCG and HCS), are produced by the syncytiotrophoblast of the human placenta. Because these hormones reflect placental rather than fetal integrity, the presence of HCG in the urine or blood may persist after fetal death (in the case of missed abortion) and even after spontaneous or therapeutic abortion. HCG is immunologically quite similar to pituitary luteinizing hormone (LH), the difference being in the amino-acid sequence of the beta subunit. This fact must be considered when interpreting results of pregnancy tests based on HCG bioassay, results of which are not always positive until 42 days gestational age. The specific immunoassay for the beta subunit of HCG, on the other hand, may be positive even before a menstrual period is missed. Progesterone is made in large amounts by the placenta. There is no good evidence to support a placental role in the production of adrenocorticosteroids.

327. The answer is A (1, 2, 3). *(Pritchard, ed 15. pp 204-210.)* Ultrasonographic visualization of the fetal head, which is generally possible by 14 weeks menstrual age, is an unmistakable sign of pregnancy. Earlier identification of the gestational "ring," which may occur at six to eight weeks, does not necessarily imply a true pregnancy, because a blighted ovum could present the same appearance. Detection of the funic (umbilical-cord) souffle is a positive sign of pregnancy, because cord pulsations are synchronous with the fetal heart beat. The uterine souffle, on the other hand, is synchronous with the maternal heart rate and does not necessarily imply pregnancy. Perception of fetal movements by an experienced examiner also is diagnostic of pregnancy. A positive urinary (or serum) chorionic gonadotropin (or beta subunit) level is not diagnostic of pregnancy; hydatidiform mole and other tumors may produce this hormone.

328. The answer is C (2, 4). *(Pritchard, ed 15. pp 480, 833.)* An infant with Potter's syndrome generally presents as a breech. After birth, the baby never is able to ventilate adequately. These infants rarely survive more than a few hours. The primary lesion in Potter's syndrome is thought to be renal. Because of renal agenesis, urine output is impossible, and oligohydramnios results. Oligohydramnios is believed to lead to pulmonary hypoplasia, because lack of amniotic fluid somehow restricts normal lung development. The characteristic facial anomalies (large, low-set ears and flattened nose) are thought to be related to pressure on the face increased by a lack of cushioning amniotic fluid. The diagnosis of Potter's syndrome has been made antenatally with the aid of ultrasonography. Demonstration of a fetal bladder that fills and empties should rule out Potter's syndrome. The absence of evidence of a bladder, despite repeated ultrasonographic examinations, would be compatible with the diagnosis. Amnion nodosum, another common finding in Potter's syndrome, consists of multiple opaque nodules in the amnion. Their etiology is not clear, but they represent fetal squames that have become "parasitic" on the membranes.

329. The answer is D (4). *(Pritchard, ed 15. pp 658-659.)* Hypertonic uterine dysfunction is characterized by a lack of coordination of uterine contractions, possibly caused by disorganization of the contraction gradient, which normally is greatest at the fundus and least at the cervix. This type of dysfunction usually appears during the latent phase of labor and is responsive to sedation, not oxytocin stimulation. The disorder is accompanied by a great deal of discomfort with little cervical dilatation (the familiar and painful "false labor"). After being sedated for a few hours, affected women usually awaken in active labor.

330. The answer is E (all). *(Pritchard, ed 15. p 663.)* Precipitate labor is labor that either is extremely rapid or is not perceived by the patient or obstetrician. For example, some women who have had presacral neurectomy do not have painful contractions and thus may be unaware they are in labor. Rapid precipitate labor, which is more common, may be due to extremely strong or prolonged contractions. Because these contractions interfere with the proper oxygenation of fetal blood, fetal hypoxia can result. Extremely strong or long contractions coupled with an unyielding cervix or vagina may predispose to amniotic fluid embolism or tears of the cervix or vagina. Sudden delivery with rapid compression and decompression of the fetal head may cause cerebral trauma.

331. The answer is E (all). *(Pritchard, ed 15. p 280.)* Ampicillin is thought to cause a reduction in urinary estriol excretion by killing certain intestinal bacteria that normally split the sulfate moiety from estriol sulfate. This bacterial reaction allows estriol to be reabsorbed from the gut and eventually excreted in the urine. Thus, the administration of ampicillin (and certain other antibiotics) may cause some estriol to be excreted in the stool rather than in the urine. Steroids may decrease estriol production by suppressing the fetal adrenal glands and reducing synthesis of estriol precursors. Maternal pyelonephritis may reduce urinary estriol content by interfering with estriol clearance by the kidneys. Placental sulfatase deficiency leads to very low urinary estriol levels, because sulfatase is essential in the conversion of sulfated estriol precursors to estriol.

332. The answer is E (all). *(Pritchard, ed 15. pp 870-871.)* Prerequisites for application of forceps include engagement, full cervical dilation, ruptured membranes, knowledge of the position of the presenting part, and fetal presentation as either vertex or face (mentum anterior). If the forceps are applied prior to engagement, trauma to maternal organs and injury to the fetus are possible. Delivery of the unengaged head should be by cesarean section. If the cervix is not fully dilated, severe cervical lacerations, including intra-abdominal trauma, may result. If the membranes are unruptured, the forceps can slip around the head. If the position of the presenting part is not established, injury to the fetus can result.

333. The answer is B (1, 3). *(Pritchard, ed 15. pp 388-389.)* The Apgar scoring system, which assesses an infant's condition one minute and five minutes after birth, is based on heart rate, respiratory effort, muscle tone, reflex irritability, and body color. The maximum score is 10 (two points per category) and the lowest score is 0. Two points are given for each of the following: a heart rate greater than 100 per minute; good respiratory effort; active motion; vigorous crying; and pink body color. A score of 0 indicates that an infant shows no response in a given category; and responses that are less than optimal but are nonetheless present earn a score of 1. Apgar scores of 4 to 7 indicate mild respiratory depression; infants who have scores under 4 are considered severely depressed. The one-minute Apgar score is best for judging the necessity of immediate resuscitation, and the five-minute Apgar score is best as an index of infant morbidity and mortality.

334. The answer is C (2, 4). *(Pritchard, ed 15. p 246.)* Describing an obstetric history by the four-digit system is more comprehensive than merely indicating parity and gravidity. The first digit of the four indicates the number of term infants delivered; the second, the number of premature infants delivered; the third, the number of abortions; and the fourth, the number of children now alive. A woman described as 7-2-1-6, therefore, has had seven term deliveries, two premature deliveries, and one abortion; and six of her children currently are alive.

335. The answer is D (4). *(Pritchard, ed 15. pp 529-531.)* Monozygotic twins are formed from the splitting of a single fertilized ovum. Dizygotic twins, which are more common, result from multiple ovulations during the same menstrual cycle. The incidence of monozygotic twinning seems to be relatively constant despite differences in race, heredity, age, and hormonal therapy. Dizygotic twinning, on the other hand, is influenced by all of these factors; it occurs more commonly in blacks than in whites, seems to run (by the maternal-hereditary line) in families, and is more common with increasing age and parity. The use of clomiphene for ovulation induction is associated with multiple ovulation and an approximately 7 percent incidence of multiple gestation (as opposed to approximately 1.0 to 1.4 percent in the normal population). The use of gonadotropins to stimulate ovulation is associated with an even higher incidence of multiple gestations, with some series reporting as high as 40 percent.

336. The answer is C (2, 4). *(Pritchard, ed 15. pp 156-157, 184-185.)* Immunoglobulin G (IgG) easily crosses the placenta and thus is found in approximately equal amounts in maternal and fetal blood. Immunoglobulin M (IgM), on the other hand, is a large molecule and does not cross the placenta. Thus maternal levels of IgM are higher than fetal levels, unless an intrauterine infection causes the fetus to manufacture IgM. The gamma chains in hemoglobin are what distinguish fetal hemoglobin from adult hemoglobin. Fetal hemoglobin (hemoglobin F) contains two alpha and two gamma chains. Hemoglobin A, found in most adults, contains two alpha and two beta chains. One would therefore expect to find more gamma chains in the fetal blood than in maternal blood. Finally, cord-blood fibrinogen levels are normally quite low; maternal fibrinogen levels, on the other hand, are about 50 percent higher than levels in nonpregnant women.

337. The answer is B (1, 3). *(Pritchard, ed 15. pp 584-588.)* Asymptomatic bacteriuria, more common during early pregnancy than late, is defined as the growth of more than 100,000 organisms of a single species in a one-milliliter, clean-voided sample of urine. The prevalence has variously been reported as low as 2 percent and as high as 12 percent; race, socioeconomic status, and parity all seem to affect the prevalence. One-fourth of women who have asymptomatic bacteriuria eventually develop acute symptomatic bacteriuria. Although bacteriuria long has been associated with premature labor, a causal relationship has not been proven, and the association may not be as significant as once thought.

338. The answer is E (all). *(Pritchard, ed 15. pp 757-764.)* The agents most responsible for puerperal infections are those normally found in the lower genital tract or in the bowel. These agents may be anaerobic bacteria (most commonly *Bacteroides, Peptostreptococcus,* and *Clostridium*) or aerobic bacteria (such as *Escherichia coli, Klebsiella, Pseudomonas,* and *Enterobacter*); infections caused by a combination of two or more pathogens occur frequently. Most puerperal infections are wound infections; trauma before or during delivery and iatrogenic bacterial contamination are significant etiologic factors. Puerperal morbidity is defined as a temperature of 38°C (100.4°F) or higher occurring on any two of the first ten postpartum days, excluding the first.

339. The answer is E (all). *(Pritchard, ed 15. p 620.)* Maternal diabetes mellitus can affect a pregnant woman and her fetus in many ways. The development of pre-eclampsia or eclampsia is about four times as likely as among nondiabetic women. Infection also is more likely not only to occur but also to be severe. The incidences of fetal macrosomia or death and of dystocia are increased; and hydramnios is common. The likelihood of postpartum hemorrhage after vaginal delivery and the frequency of cesarean section both are increased in diabetic women.

340. The answer is D (4). *(Pritchard, ed 15. p 281.)* The oxytocin challenge test assesses the ability of the fetoplacental unit to withstand the stress of labor. After external monitors have measured the baseline activity of the uterus and fetal heart for ten minutes, intravenous oxytocin is infused at a rate of 0.5 milliunits per minute. The rate is doubled every 15 to 20 minutes until three contractions, that each last for 40 to 60 seconds, occur every ten minutes. The test is considered positive if fetal heart rate consistently decelerates once uterine contractions have begun.

341. The answer is A (1, 2, 3). *(Pritchard, ed 15. pp 680-690.)* Shoulder presentation, either as a transverse or an oblique lie, presents significant problems when vaginal delivery of an affected infant is attempted. Similarly, persistent brow presentation and the presence of a prolapsed umbilical cord also are associated with significant compromise of infants delivered vaginally. Persistent occiput posterior position does not significantly compromise an infant during the course of a normal vaginal delivery.

342. The answer is B (1, 3). *(Pritchard, ed 15. pp 744-748.)* The most common causes of immediate postpartum hemorrhage are uterine atony and vaginal or cervical lacerations. Retained placental fragments may be responsible for delayed postpartum bleeding but rarely cause immediate hemorrhage. An exception might be if a succenturiate lobe of the placenta were left within the uterus. Congenital anomalies of the uterus are not known to cause postpartum hemorrhage.

343. The answer is C (2, 4). *(Pritchard, ed 15. pp 184-185, 190, 195.)* Plasma fibrinogen levels increase about 50 percent during pregnancy. This rise is thought to be at least partially responsible for the great increase in the erythrocyte sedimentation rate. The elevated sedimentation rate is consequently almost useless as a significant laboratory value in pregnant women. Serum albumin decreases by almost one-third during normal pregnancy. Blood urea nitrogen (BUN) decreases markedly during pregnancy; in fact, BUN values falling in the mid-normal range for nonpregnant women (around 10 mg/100 ml) may signal significant impairment of renal function in pregnant women.

344-348. The answers are: 344-D, 345-C, 346-C, 347-B, 348-E. *(Pritchard, ed 15. pp 406-407, 416-417, 433, 487, 749.)* Placenta previa is characterized by defective vascularization of the decidua, secondary to either inflammatory or atrophic changes; in this uncommon condition, the placenta is implanted over or near the internal os. Abruptio placentae (placental abruption), which is associated very closely with maternal hypertension, is the premature separation of the placenta from the uterus. The Arias-Stella phenomenon, which refers to certain changes of the glands and epithelium of the endometrium, frequently is associated with ectopic pregnancy; however, this phenomenon also can occur whenever a conceptus is blighted and may be seen in intrauterine as well as extrauterine pregnancies. Spontaneous abortions histologically are accompanied by distended placental villi, hemorrhage into the decidua basalis, and evidence of necrotic changes in the region surrounding the hemorrhage.

349-351. The answers are: 349-D, 350-A, 351-B. *(Pritchard, ed 15. pp 288, 871, 899-901, 905-906.)* A woman who has been at 9 cm for 3 hours is experiencing a secondary arrest in labor. Deteriorating fetal condition (as evidenced, for example, by late decelerations and falling scalp pH) dictates immediate delivery. A forceps rotation would be inappropriate, because the cervix is not fully dilated. Cesarean section would be the safest and most expeditious method. Classical cesarean section is rarely used now because of greater blood loss and a higher incidence in subsequent pregnancies of rupture of the scar prior to labor. The best procedure would be a low transverse cesarean section.

A transverse lie is undeliverable. One treatment option is to do nothing and hope that the lie will be longitudinal by the time labor commences. The only other appropriate maneuver would be to perform an external cephalic version. This maneuver should be done in the hospital, with monitoring of the fetal heart. If the version is successful and the cervix is ripe, it might be best to take advantage of the favorable vertex position by rupturing the membranes at that point and inducing labor.

Diagnosing twins at the time of delivery is not at all unusual, happening as often as 50 percent of the time, according to some studies. This statistic may no longer be true in those centers using ultrasound examination on a routine basis. The second twin is probably the only remaining situation where internal version is permissible. Although some obstetricians might perform a cesarean section for a second twin presenting as a footling or shoulder, fetal bradycardia dictates that immediate delivery be done; and internal podalic version is the quickest procedure.

352-354. The answers are: 352-B, 353-D, 354-A. *(Pritchard, ed 15. pp 231-232.)* The four general pelvic configurations, named here according to the widely used Caldwell-Moloy classification, may be important indicators of potential problems during labor and delivery. The gynecoid pelvis, the most common type, is generally round, with the transverse diameter being the same as or slightly greater than the anteroposterior diameter.

The anthropoid pelvis is essentially oblong, with the anteroposterior diameter being much greater than the transverse diameter. It is thus a deep, narrow pelvis; characteristically, the ischial spines are prominent and the sacrum is inclined posteriorly.

The android pelvis is often described as triangular. The anterior pelvis is narrowed, with a narrow subpubic angle; but, unlike the anthropoid pelvis, the posterior pelvis is short, with a small posterior sagittal diameter. The spines are prominent in the android pelvis, and the sacrum is straight. Unless it is unusually large, this type of pelvis offers a poor prognosis for delivery.

The rarest pelvic type is the platypelloid ("flat") pelvis. Here the anteroposterior diameter is quite short and the transverse diameter is wide. The subpubic angle is wide and the ischial spines are not prominent. This type of pelvis may cause the vertex to stay in the occiput transverse position until delivery.

355-358. The answers are: 355-A, 356-C, 357-A, 358-B. *(Pritchard, ed 15. pp 151-153.)* Oxygen travels from mother to fetus, and carbon dioxide from fetus to mother, by simple diffusion across the placenta. Carbon dioxide travels more rapidly than oxygen, probably because fetal and maternal blood have different affinities for these two substances. Iron is actively transported (i.e., in an energy-requiring process) from mother to fetus; as a result, the mother may become markedly iron-depleted during pregnancy, while the fetus does well. Glucose crosses to the fetus by facilitated diffusion, which means that its transfer across the placenta is more rapid than could be accounted for by simple diffusion alone. The fetus acts as a "glucose sink," continuously obtaining glucose at the expense of the mother. This fact may help to explain the lower-than-normal levels of maternal fasting blood glucose found during pregnancy.

359-363. The answers are: 359-C, 360-E, 361-A, 362-E, 363-B. *(Pritchard, ed 15. p 258.)* The recommendations concerning immunization during pregnancy offered by the American College of Obstetricians and Gynecologists are as follows:

--Administration of influenza vaccine is recommended if the underlying disease is serious;

--Typhoid immunization is recommended when traveling to an endemic region;

--Hepatitis-A immunization is recommended after exposure or before travel to developing countries;

--Cholera immunization should be given only to meet travel requirements;

--Tetanus-diphtheria immunization should be given if a primary series has never been administered or if ten years have elapsed without receiving a booster;

--Immunization for poliomyelitis is mandatory during an epidemic but otherwise not recommended;

--Smallpox immunization should be avoided except in the event of probable exposure;

--Immunization for yellow fever is contraindicated unless exposure is unavoidable;

--Mumps and rubella immunization is contraindicated; and

--Administration of rabies vaccine is unaffected by pregnancy.

364-366. The answers are: 364-C, 365-B, 366-E. *(Pritchard, ed 15. pp 468-474, 749-751.)* A circumvallate placenta contains a grayish-white ring located a variable distance from the edge of the placenta. The membranes (amnion and chorion) are folded over at this ring and are not in contact with the substance of the placenta peripheral to the ring. The fetal vessels do not go beyond the ring. Placenta circumvallata is associated with an increased rate of prematurity; why the rate is increased is unknown.

A succenturiate placenta is characterized by an accessory lobe apart from the main body of the placenta. Fetal vessels usually course through the membranes between the main and accessory lobes and can be identified on inspection of the membranes. If the fetal vessels on their way between the lobes should pass over the cervix, vasa praevia occurs. This condition is potentially dangerous, because the membranes may rupture, in turn rupturing a fetal vessel and causing fetal hemorrhage. If a succenturiate lobe is left within the uterus after the main body of the placenta has been delivered, postpartum hemorrhage can result; therefore, the presence of an accessory lobe should be checked for by intrauterine exploration.

Placenta accreta is a condition in which the usual plane of cleavage (Nitabuch's layer) between the placenta and decidua is absent and the villi attach to the myometrium. It is more common in women who have uterine scars, such as in the described patient, and who had undergone previous cesarean section. Complications of placenta accreta are in part iatrogenic. A too-vigorous attempt at manual removal may cause uterine inversion or perforation and severe bleeding. A hysterectomy may be necessary, although leaving the placenta in place and treating the patient with methotrexate may suffice. Severe complications are most common with the more severe forms of placenta accreta. These forms are known as placenta increta, if the villi grow into the muscle of the uterus, and placenta percreta, if the placenta grows through the myometrium.

367-369. The answers are: 367-C, 368-B, 369-A. *(Pritchard, ed 15. pp 866-888.)* Barton forceps are designed for a transverse arrest in a platypelloid (flat) pelvis. The pelvic curve of the forceps is in an appropriate position vis-à-vis the maternal pelvis when the forceps are applied to the occiput transverse. Descent is then accomplished in this position, and rotation to the occiput anterior does not occur until the pelvic floor is reached. Rotation in the midplane thus is unnecessary; indeed, such rotation would be difficult in a flat pelvis.

Kielland's forceps are designed specifically for rotation. They have very little pelvic curve and thus are unlikely to cause maternal soft tissue injury during rotation. They can be used for occiput posterior or transverse positions, in which rotation is planned before traction is applied.

Simpson's forceps are the prototype forceps for the molded head. They are useful for low forceps deliveries; and some obstetricians use Simpson's or similar forceps for various rotation maneuvers.

Chamberlen forceps were probably the first true obstetric forceps, in use by the late sixteenth century. Tarnier's forceps are also of historical interest. They were used to effect extremely difficult deliveries in situations that today generally would call for cesarean section.

Obstetrics and Gynecology

Infectious Disease

Ronald S. Gibbs

DIRECTIONS: Each question below contains five suggested answers. Choose the **one best** response to each question.

370. In a pregnant woman who has had prolonged, premature rupture of the fetal membranes, the earliest sign of chorioamnionitis would be

(A) maternal fever
(B) maternal leukocytosis
(C) maternal tachycardia
(D) fetal tachycardia
(E) a foul odor to the amniotic fluid

Questions 371-372

A woman develops endometritis after a cesarean section has been performed. She is treated with penicillin and gentamicin but fails to respond.

371. Which of the following bacteria is resistant to these antibiotics and is likely to be responsible for this woman's infection?

(A) *Proteus mirabilis*
(B) *Bacteroides fragilis*
(C) *Escherichia coli*
(D) Alpha streptococci
(E) Anaerobic streptococci

372. The antibiotic of choice for treating this woman would be

(A) polymyxin
(B) ampicillin
(C) cephalothin
(D) vancomycin
(E) clindamycin

373. A pregnant woman is discovered to be an asymptomatic carrier of *Neisseria gonorrhoeae*. A year ago, she was treated with penicillin for a gonococcal infection and developed a severe allergic reaction. Treatment of choice at this time would be

(A) tetracycline
(B) ampicillin
(C) erythromycin
(D) spectinomycin
(E) chloramphenicol

374. Cytomegalovirus, which can cause severe intrauterine infection, can be recovered from the cervices of approximately what percentage of women in the United States?

(A) 0.005 percent
(B) 0.05 percent
(C) 0.5 percent
(D) 5 percent
(E) 50 percent

375. At term, a pregnant woman has herpesvirus hominis (herpes simplex) type 2 lesions on her vulva and vagina. What is the chance that her infant will develop an infection after delivery?

(A) 0.5 percent
(B) 1 percent
(C) 5 percent
(D) 30 percent
(E) 75 percent

376. A 19-year-old nulliparous woman is given a Venereal Disease Research Laboratories (VDRL) test, which is positive at a dilution of 1:4. The diagnostic measure that now should be ordered is a

(A) Wasserman-type test
(B) rapid plasma reagin card test
(C) fluorescent treponemal antibody-absorption (FTA-ABS) test
(D) lumbar puncture and VDRL titer of cerebrospinal fluid
(E) thorough pelvic examination

DIRECTIONS: Each question below contains four suggested answers of which **one** or **more** is correct. Choose the answer:

A	if	**1, 2, and 3**	are correct
B	if	**1 and 3**	are correct
C	if	**2 and 4**	are correct
D	if	**4**	is correct
E	if	**1, 2, 3, and 4**	are correct

377. A pregnant woman (12 weeks) undergoes an outpatient suction abortion. She returns three days later with a temperature of 39.2°C (102.5°F), lower abdominal cramps, and vaginal bleeding. The uterus is boggy on examination. Appropriate therapy should include

(1) culture and Gram stain of the endocervix
(2) culture of venous blood
(3) antibiotic therapy
(4) uterine curettage

378. A young primigravid woman is found to have asymptomatic *Escherichia coli* bacteriuria at her first prenatal visit. Which of the following statements about this woman are true?

(1) She is clearly at risk for delivering prematurely
(2) She is clearly at risk for developing pyelonephritis
(3) She is clearly at risk for developing toxemia of pregnancy
(4) She should be treated with oral antibiotics

379. A Gram stain of pus taken from a tubo-ovarian abscess reveals gram-positive cocci. Penicillin G is the drug of choice for all such organisms EXCEPT

(1) group A, beta-hemolytic streptococci
(2) *Streptococcus faecalis* (enterococci)
(3) anaerobic streptococci
(4) *Staphylococcus aureus*

380. A 68-year-old woman, who is receiving chemotherapy for metastatic ovarian carcinoma, develops sepsis, for which bacteriocidal antibiotics are indicated. Which of the following antibiotics are bacteriocidal?

(1) Penicillin
(2) Tetracycline
(3) Cephalothin
(4) Chloramphenicol

381. A young woman develops painful vulvar vesicles, and a herpesvirus hominis (herpes simplex) infection is suspected. What tests can be done to confirm this diagnosis?

(1) Wet mount with saline
(2) Culture for the virus
(3) Gram stain
(4) Papanicolaou smear

382. Which of the following conditions predispose to vaginal infection with *Candida albicans*?

(1) Pregnancy
(2) Antibiotic therapy
(3) Adrenocorticosteroid therapy
(4) Presence of an intrauterine device

383. Chorioamnionitis develops in a woman whose membranes have ruptured at 35 weeks gestation; the fetus is alive. Management should include

(1) systemic antibiotics
(2) high-dose corticosteroids
(3) delivery by either a brief induction or cesarean section
(4) heparinization

384. A 27-year-old woman has an increased vaginal discharge, lower abdominal pain, and a low-grade fever; a neisserial infection is suspected. Appropriate culture media for the identification of *Neisseria gonorrhoeae* from the cervix include

(1) thioglycollate broth
(2) blood agar in a candle jar
(3) blood agar in an anaerobic chamber
(4) Thayer-Martin medium in a candle jar

385. The differential diagnosis of acute gonorrheal salpingitis includes which of the following disorders?

(1) Septic abortion
(2) Ectopic pregnancy
(3) Acute appendicitis
(4) Ruptured ovarian cyst

386. Following a vaginal delivery, a woman develops a fever, lower abdominal pain, and uterine tenderness. She is alert, and her blood pressure and urine output are good. Large gram-positive rods suggestive of *Clostridia* are seen in a smear of the cervix. Management should include

(1) close observation for renal failure or hemolysis
(2) immediate radiographic examination for gas in the uterus
(3) high-dose antibiotic therapy
(4) hysterectomy

387. The use of which of the following antibiotics is contraindicated during pregnancy?

(1) Tetracycline
(2) Penicillin
(3) Chloramphenicol
(4) Ampicillin

DIRECTIONS: The groups of questions below consist of lettered choices followed by several numbered items. For each numbered item select the **one** lettered choice with which it is **most** closely associated. Each lettered choice may be used once, more than once, or not at all.

Questions 388-391

For each description that follows, select the microorganism with which it is most likely to be associated.

(A) Rubella virus
(B) Cytomegalovirus
(C) Group A beta-hemolytic streptococci
(D) Group B beta-hemolytic streptococci
(E) *Toxoplasma gondii*

388. This organism may cause epidemics of puerperal sepsis

389. A pregnant woman may become infected with this organism by contact with infected cat feces

390. An effective vaccine exists for the prevention of adult infection with this organism

391. This organism is an important cause of neonatal sepsis and meningitis

Questions 392-395

For each description that follows, select the antibiotic with which it is most likely to be associated.

(A) Gentamicin
(B) Ampicillin
(C) Tetracycline
(D) Cephalothin
(E) A sulfonamide antibiotic

392. A 23-year-old woman who has had a septic abortion has positive blood cultures with an organism that is identified as an aerobic gram-negative rod; this antibiotic would be the drug of choice

393. A 73-year-old woman has a urinary tract infection with *Escherichia coli*; because she refuses an injection and insists on oral medication, this antibiotic should **not** be administered

394. This antibiotic is the drug of choice for treating nonpregnant women who have *Mycoplasma hominis* infections

395. This antibiotic may be used in early pregnancy but is contraindicated after 32 weeks of gestation

Obstetrics and Gynecology

Infectious Disease

Answers

370. The answer is D. *(Monif, p 297.)* Fetal tachycardia in a woman who has had prolonged, premature rupture of fetal membranes strongly suggests chorioamnionitis, which can be confirmed by stain and culture of amniotic fluid. Maternal fever and leukocytosis are later signs of infection. The presence of fetal tachycardia should be interpreted with caution, however, because it also can arise as a result of an arrhythmia or exposure to drugs, such as atropine.

371. The answer is B. *(Monif, pp 8, 439-441.)* Infections caused by *Bacteroides fragilis*, a gram-negative anaerobic bacillus, are a significant obstetric problem. Not only is the organism resistant to many commonly used antibiotics (including penicillin and gentamicin), but it is difficult to isolate, culture, and identify as well. The high incidence of gynecologic and obstetric *B. fragilis* infections may be due to the pathogen's predominance among the anaerobic bacteria of the lower bowel. Although the other organisms listed in the question also can cause postpartum infection, they are sensitive to antibiotic therapy with penicillin and gentamicin.

372. The answer is E. *(Monif, pp 8, 441-442.)* Clindamycin is the most effective antibiotic for treating women who have bacteroidosis. Chloramphenicol and tetracycline are alternative choices for antibiotic therapy in nonpregnant women; however, tetracycline-resistant strains of *Bacteroides fragilis* may be emerging. Lincomycin and erythromycin also can be effective in the management of affected women.

373. The answer is C. *(Monif, p 8.)* Erythromycin is the treatment of choice for pregnant women who have an asymptomatic *Neisseria gonorrhoeae* infection and who are allergic to penicillin. Although tetracycline also is an effective alternative to pencillin, its use is contraindicated in pregnancy. Spectinomycin is another drug effective in treating asymptomatic gonorrhea, but erythromycin is preferred in pregnant women because of uncertain effects of spectinomycin on the fetus. Administration of chloramphenicol is not recommended to treat women, pregnant or not, who have cervical gonorrhea, and the use of ampicillin is contraindicated for penicillin-allergic patients.

374. The answer is D. *(Monif, p 43.)* Cytomegalovirus is found in 3 to 6 percent of endocervical cultures of American women. However, unlike herpesvirus, the presence of cytomegalovirus in the cervix does not pose a major threat to the fetus passing through the genital canal. Cytomegalovirus can cause a severe intrauterine infection, however, if viremia results in a transplacental infection.

375. The answer is D. *(Nahmias, Am J Obstet Gynecol 110[1971]:825.)* Herpesvirus hominis type 2 infection is highly contagious and develops in 20 to at least 40 percent of all neonates delivered vaginally from women who have herpetic vulvovaginitis. These neonatal infections are usually fulminant and are associated with a mortality rate of more than 60 percent. Neurologic or ocular disease affects most of the survivors.

376. The answer is C. *(Monif, pp 176-177.)* Because a positive VDRL test either may indicate the presence of syphilis or may be a biologic false positive, a specific treponemal test, such as the fluorescent treponemal antibody-absorption (FTA-ABS) test, is needed to discriminate false positives from true infection. The rapid plasma reagin (RPR) card test and Wasserman-type tests, such as the Kolmer test, are nontreponemal tests and therefore are no more specific than the VDRL test. A lumbar puncture would not be indicated at this point. A pelvic examination may be of little diagnostic use, because chancres often disappear before a VDRL test becomes positive.

377. The answer is E (all). *(Monif, pp 278-280.)* Culture and Gram stain of the endocervix are important in directing antibiotic therapy for women who have had septic abortions. Blood cultures also can be very helpful, because they are positive in 30 to 50 percent of patients who have an abortion-related infection. Broad-spectrum antibiotic therapy is, of course, indicated. Moreover, in a woman who has a fever, cramps, and vaginal bleeding following an abortion, retention of conception products must be suspected, and curettage should be performed.

378. The answer is C (2, 4). *(Monif, pp 322-323.)* Women who have asymptomatic bacteriuria have a 20 to 30 percent chance of developing pyelonephritis and therefore should be treated with oral antibiotics. Most cases of pyelonephritis of pregnancy could be prevented by treating asymptomatic bacteriuria. The relationship between asymptomatic bacteriuria and other complications, such as premature labor and toxemia of pregnancy, has been suggested but not clearly established.

379. The answer is C (2, 4). *(Monif, pp 8-9.)* *Streptococcus faecalis* (enterococci), which is commonly resistant to penicillin G alone, is sensitive either to ampicillin or to a synergistic combination of pencillin G and an aminoglycoside (such as streptomycin, kanamycin, or gentamicin). Approximately 85 to 95 percent of species of *Staphylococcus aureus* produce penicillinase and thus are resistant to penicillin G; other antibiotics that are effective against this organism include cephalosporin, vancomycin, and erythromycin.

380. The answer is B (1, 3). *(Monif, p 6.)* Penicillin and cephalothin are bacteriocidal antibiotics that interfere with bacterial cell-wall synthesis. Tetracycline and chloramphenicol, which are bacteriostatic antibiotics, interfere with protein synthesis.

381. The answer is C (2, 4). *(Monif, p 56.)* Herpesvirus hominis (herpes simplex) can be cultured readily and rapidly; however, available facilities to perform viral cultures are limited. A Pap smear will show typical herpetic findings (multinucleated giant cells and intranuclear inclusions) in approximately 85 percent of affected women. Wet mounts and Gram stains are inadequate detectors of viral infection.

382. The answer is A (1, 2, 3). *(Monif, pp 242-243.)* Pregnancy is associated with an increase in the incidence of monilial infections, probably because of an increase in glycogen content in the vaginal mucosa. Antibiotic therapy clearly increases the likelihood of candidiasis (moniliasis), perhaps because it eliminates susceptible bacteria that compete with *Candida* for available nutrients. Steroid therapy also increases the likelihood of candidiasis; the mechanism of action may involve inhibition of catabolic-enzyme release. No association exists between the use of intrauterine devices and a predisposition toward monilial infections.

383. The answer is B (1, 3). *(Monif, pp 297-299.)* The main mode of treatment for women who have chorioamnionitis is delivery. If the cervix is effaced and dilated, a brief induction could be undertaken; if the cervix is unripe, then abdominal delivery would be in order. Administration of potent antibiotics is important to prevent the mother from developing sepsis. Although corticosteroids are not indicated in the treatment of women who have uncomplicated chorioamnionitis, such therapy might be valuable if septic shock develops. The use of steroids to accelerate pulmonary maturity would be inappropriate. Heparinization is not indicated in uncomplicated chorioamnionitis. Coagulation disorders, which may be a complication of severe infection, should not be treated unless there is uncontrollable bleeding.

384. The answer is D (4). *(Monif, pp 390-391.)* Selective media must be used for the identification of *Neisseria gonorrhoeae* taken from the genital tract. Cultures using nonselective media are likely to be overgrown with other pelvic bacteria. Culturing multiple sites, especially the anus and oropharynx, in addition to the cervix, can result in the detection of approximately 90 percent of gonorrheal infections in women; multiple-site culturing is best used as a means of monitoring the effectiveness of treatment.

385. The answer is E (all). *(Monif, p 391.)* The differential diagnosis of acute gonorrheal salpingitis is extensive and includes many other causes of lower abdominal pain. Disorders that must be included in the differential diagnosis are septic abortion, ectopic pregnancy, acute appendicitis, torsion of adnexal structures, and ruptured ovarian cyst.

386. The answer is A (1, 2, 3). *(Monif, pp 435-438.)* *Clostridia* can be seen in 5 to 10 percent of pelvic cultures. When the organism is found, appropriate antibiotic therapy (e.g., with penicillin) and close observation for gas gangrene, hemolysis, and renal failure are in order. Presumed identification on the basis of Gram stain alone or the presence of a mild infection without signs of sepsis or extrauterine involvement are not reason enough to proceed to hysterectomy.

387. The answer is B (1, 3). *(Monif, pp 19-26.)* Tetracycline may cause fetal dental anomalies and inhibition of bone growth if administered during the second trimester, and it is a potential teratogen to first-trimester fetuses. Tetracycline administration also can cause severe hepatic decompensation in the mother, especially during the third trimester. Chloramphenicol may cause the "gray baby" syndrome (symptoms of which include vomiting, impaired respiration, hypothermia, and, finally, cardiovascular collapse) in neonates who have received large doses of the drug. No notable adverse effects have been associated with the use of penicillin or ampicillin.

388-391. The answers are: 388-C, 389-E, 390-A, 391-D. *(Monif, pp 73, 197-198, 306, 455.)* Group A beta-hemolytic streptococci can cause puerperal or postoperative pelvic infection. Outbreaks of puerperal fever are still reported on obstetric services, though not at anywhere near the frequency of 50 years ago. When the disease does occur, a point source among the hospital personnel should be suspected.

Group B beta-hemolytic streptococci, which also can cause puerperal fever, have recently been recognized as a major cause of severe neonatal infection. The organism can be isolated from about 5 percent of the cervices of pregnant women; infection of the infant, which can result in sepsis, occurs as the infant passes through the vagina.

Toxoplasma gondii, a protozoan parasite, is transmitted by flies from cat feces to human food. Humans thus can become infected by consuming infected meat that is inadequately cooked or by directly contacting feces of an infected cat. Acute toxoplasmosis in a pregnant woman may cause a fulminant fetal infection; infected neonates may be born with microcephaly, intracranial calcification, or other symptoms.

An effective attenuated-virus vaccine is available for immunization against rubella. However, its use is contraindicated for pregnant women and commonly is associated with development of arthralgia in adults.

392-395. The answers are: 392-A, 393-A, 394-C, 395-E. *(Monif, pp 9, 26, 159.)* Gentamicin, an aminoglycoside similar to kanamycin and streptomycin, is not absorbed after oral administration. It is the drug of choice for women who have severe infections caused by gram-negative aerobes. Although *Mycoplasma hominis* commonly is found in the genital tract, its role in producing infections is unclear. Documented mycoplasmal infections are best treated with tetracycline, except if the affected woman is pregnant. Sulfonamide administration is contraindicated in late pregnancy. Because this antibiotic crosses the placenta and competes with bilirubin for binding sites in the fetus, it can lead to hyperbilirubinemia and kernicterus in the neonate.

Perinatology
General Considerations

Richard L. Berkowitz

Donald R. Coustan

DIRECTIONS: Each question below contains five suggested answers. Choose the **one best** response to each question.

396. A woman who has adult-onset (class B) diabetes requires an elective cesarean section. Her diabetes has been well controlled throughout the pregnancy and she has had normal uterine growth. Her first antepartum visit was at 18 weeks. Weekly oxytocin challenge tests and daily urinary estriol determinations have been within normal limits. It has been decided that the cesarean section should be performed at 38 weeks. Which of the following tests would provide the most useful information on the day prior to the procedure?

(A) Fasting blood glucose
(B) Fetal biparietal diameter
(C) Radiographic study of fetal femoral epiphyses
(D) Lecithin-sphingomyelin ratio
(E) Amniotic fluid alpha-fetoprotein level

397. All of the following conditions are known to be associated with clinically evident coagulopathies EXCEPT

(A) retained dead fetus
(B) severe pre-eclampsia
(C) sepsis
(D) intra-amniotic prostaglandin $F_{2\alpha}$ abortion
(E) amniotic fluid embolism

398. Which of the following statements describes rupture of a classic cesarean section scar in pregnant women?

(A) It can be prevented by delivery by cesarean section
(B) It is much less likely to occur than rupture of a lower-segment scar
(C) One-third of ruptures occur before the onset of labor
(D) Perinatal mortality rate is 10 percent
(E) Maternal mortality rate approaches 15 percent

399. Which of the following statements concerning placenta previa is true?

(A) Bleeding is usually painful
(B) The initial hemorrhage is rarely fatal
(C) Modern management no longer includes a "double set-up"
(D) Its incidence is unaffected by parity
(E) Its incidence decreases with maternal age

---

400. Heart tones could not be detected from a fetus at 22 weeks of gestation. Amniography was ordered, and the x-ray shown below was obtained. The diagnosis is

(A) hydatidiform mole
(B) normal intrauterine pregnancy
(C) ovarian cystadenocarcinoma
(D) abdominal pregnancy
(E) pseudocyesis

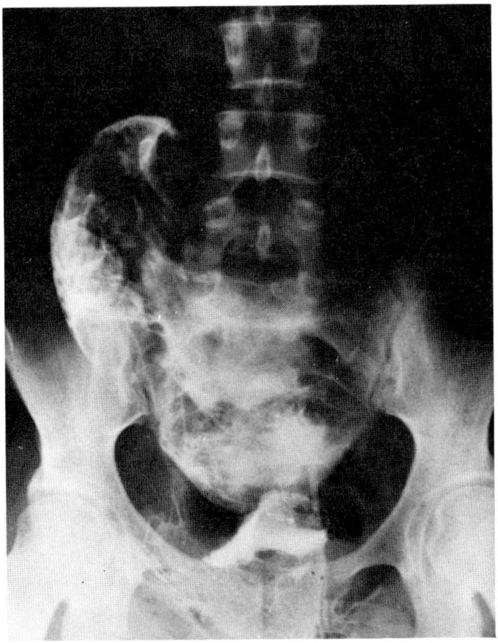

401. As pregnancy progresses, which of the following hematologic changes occurs?

(A) Plasma volume increases proportionally more than red cell volume
(B) Red cell volume increases proportionally more than plasma volume
(C) Plasma volume increases and red cell volume remains constant
(D) Red cell volume decreases and plasma volume remains constant
(E) Neither plasma volume nor red cell volume changes

402. Clinical studies have demonstrated which of the following blood pressure changes in the second trimester of pregnancy (as compared to the beginning of pregnancy)?

(A) Systolic and diastolic blood pressures both are significantly reduced
(B) Systolic blood pressure is reduced, but diastolic blood pressure is relatively unchanged
(C) Systolic blood pressure is relatively unchanged, but diastolic blood pressure is reduced
(D) Systolic blood pressure is increased, but diastolic blood pressure is relatively unchanged
(E) Systolic and diastolic blood pressures both are significantly increased

403. Which of the following statements is NOT true of renal function in normal pregnancy?

(A) Caliceal, renal pelvic, and ureteral dilatation can occur as early as the second trimester
(B) Hormonal and mechanical factors have been implicated as causes of ureteral dilatation in the third trimester
(C) Glomerular filtration rate increases about 50 percent over values in nonpregnant women
(D) Renal plasma flow increases about 35 percent over values in nonpregnant women
(E) Creatinine clearance is an accurate reflection of glomerular filtration rate during pregnancy

404. A 28-year-old primigravid woman first registers for prenatal care at 36 weeks gestation. A tuberculin skin (PPD) test is positive. The woman states she has never had a PPD test before. A chest x-ray is ordered, but the woman does not keep her appointment and, in fact, does not return to the hospital until labor has begun at 41 weeks. A chest x-ray at this time reveals minimal tuberculous changes. The woman is kept in the hospital until all of the cultures for acid-fast bacilli are reported to be negative. She is started on isoniazid (INH) chemotherapy. Appropriate treatment of the neonate would include

(A) isolation from the mother for three to six weeks
(B) administration of isoniazid
(C) vaccination with BCG vaccine
(D) a PPD test every three to four months
(E) none of the above

405. The most common cause of death in women who have eclampsia is

(A) ruptured liver
(B) acute renal failure
(C) cerebral hemorrhage
(D) pulmonary embolism
(E) septic shock

406. Beta sympathomimetic drugs, which can inhibit uterine activity, include all of the following EXCEPT

(A) salbutamol
(B) ritodrine
(C) propranolol
(D) terbutaline
(E) fenoterol

407. The initial maternal immunologic response to a primary rubella infection is the elaboration of

(A) immunoglobulin M
(B) immunoglobulin G
(C) immunoglobulin A
(D) immunoglobulin D
(E) complement-fixation antibodies

408. The x-ray shown below reveals which of the following?

(A) Hydrocephaly
(B) Term pregnancy with a dermoid cyst
(C) Fetus papyraceus
(D) Anencephaly
(E) Normal breech presentation

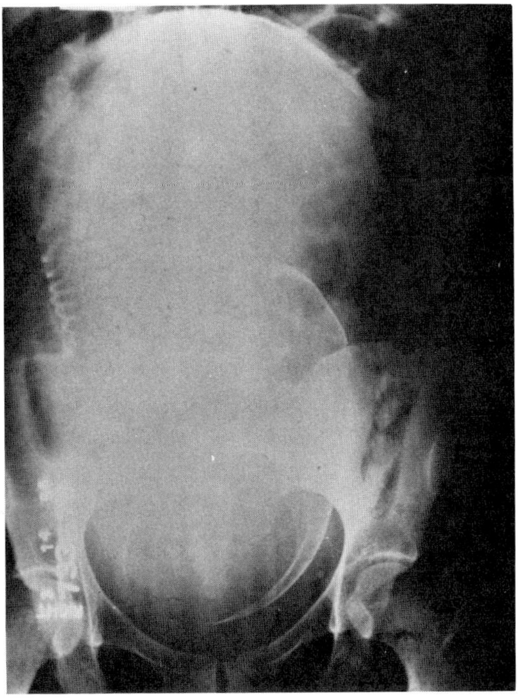

409. A pregnant woman is seen 18 days after she has been exposed to rubella. Her hemagglutination inhibition (HAI) titer is 1:8. Her physician should

(A) administer rubella vaccine
(B) recommend an abortion
(C) repeat the titer two days later
(D) repeat the titer 10 to 14 days later
(E) obtain weekly titers for the next four weeks

410. A syndrome of multiple congenital anomalies, including microcephaly, cardiac anomalies, and growth retardation, has been described in children of women who are heavy users of

(A) heroin
(B) methadone
(C) ethyl alcohol
(D) amphetamines
(E) barbiturates

411. Achondroplasia can be characterized by which of the following statements?

(A) The inheritance pattern is autosomal recessive
(B) Mutation accounts for 80 percent of all cases
(C) Cesarean section is rarely necessary
(D) Affected women rarely live to the reproductive age
(E) None of the above

412. Which of the following statements concerning the effects of smoking during pregnancy is NOT supported by epidemiologic or clinical studies?

(A) There is a reduction in birth weight of the offspring of smokers when compared to matched controls
(B) The incidence of premature labor is not increased significantly in women who smoke
(C) The incidence of toxemia of pregnancy is increased in women who smoke
(D) The effects of smoking are directly proportional to the number of cigarettes smoked
(E) The number of cigarettes smoked daily after the third month of gestation are more important than the number smoked before that time

413. Planimetric studies of the placenta support which of the following statements?

(A) The average surface area at term is 2 to 6 square meters in a normal pregnancy
(B) The average surface area at term is 11 to 14 square meters in a normal pregnancy
(C) Total capillary area is always proportional to surface area
(D) No correlation exists between surface area and functional capacity
(E) The diagnostic value of planimetric studies is significant

414. The relationship between fetal, placental, and maternal endocrine systems is characterized by

(A) identical enzymatic capabilities
(B) the addition of sulfate radicals in the placental compartment
(C) placental conversion of C-21 compounds to C-19 compounds
(D) the principal conversion of dehydroepiandrosterone sulfate to estrogens by the maternal compartment
(E) none of the above

415. Which of the following statements characterizes the estrogen present in maternal urine?

(A) Its concentration is decreased during pregnancy
(B) At term, it is 80 to 85 percent estriol
(C) At term, it is 50 percent estradiol
(D) Its excretion is normal at term in patients who have placental sulfatase deficiency
(E) Its excretion is unrelated to fetal adrenal or hepatic function

416. Viremia and the presence of rubella virus in the throat of infected individuals bear which of the following relationships to the onset of the rubella rash?

(A) They precede the rash by five to seven days
(B) They precede the rash by one to two days
(C) They occur coincidentally with the rash
(D) They occur one to two days after the rash
(E) They bear no consistent relationship to the onset of the rash

417. All of the following drugs can cross the placenta easily EXCEPT

(A) digoxin
(B) phenobarbital
(C) heparin
(D) mepivacaine
(E) tetracycline

418. A 32-year-old woman at term develops a clinically obvious coagulopathy following a classical episode of abruptio placentae. Fibrinogen concentrate should NOT be ordered for this woman because

(A) it is commercially unavailable
(B) it carries an unacceptable risk of hepatitis
(C) it increases the risk of hepatic subcapsular hemorrhage
(D) the patient's primary requirement is platelets
(E) the primary objective should be to stop fibrinolysis

419. Which line on the echogram shown below represents the biparietal diameter of the fetal skull?

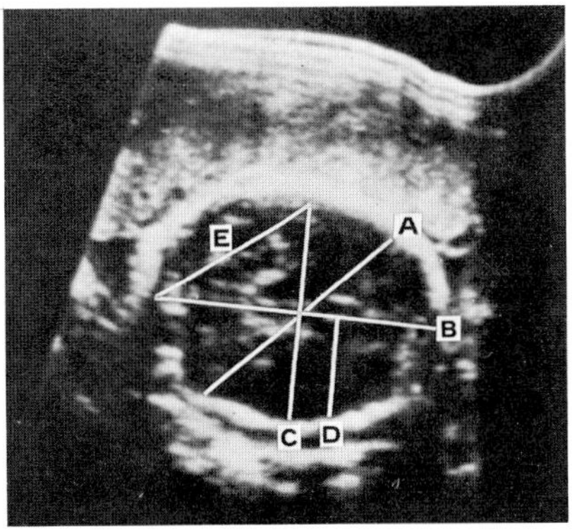

(A) Line A
(B) Line B
(C) Line C
(D) Line D
(E) Line E

420. During labor, deceleration of the fetal heart rate correlates most closely with which of the following fetal values?

(A) Arterial pH
(B) Arterial P_{O_2}
(C) Arterial P_{CO_2}
(D) Central venous pressure
(E) Venous potassium levels

421. Late deceleration patterns (Type II dips) on a fetal monitoring strip represent

(A) cord compression
(B) pulmonary immaturity
(C) fetal hypoxia secondary to decreased perfusion of the intervillous spaces
(D) congenital cardiac conduction defects
(E) entry of the fetal head into the pelvic brim

---

422. The fetal monitoring strip shown below demonstrates which of the following?

(A) A classic uteroplacental insufficiency pattern
(B) A cord pattern
(C) Head compression
(D) Uneventful labor
(E) Fetal death

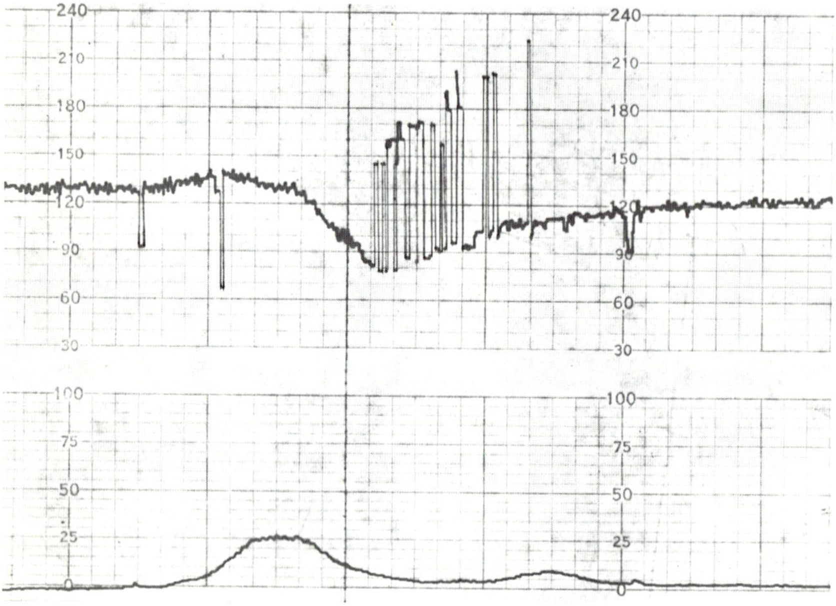

423. Although rheumatic heart disease is becoming less common, it still occurs during pregnancy. Deteriorating cardiac status in a pregnant woman is most likely to be associated with

(A) aortic regurgitation
(B) aortic stenosis
(C) mitral regurgitation
(D) mitral stenosis
(E) tricuspid regurgitation

424. The safe upper limit of traction forces to the head during a forceps delivery is

(A) 5 pounds
(B) 20 pounds
(C) 35 pounds
(D) 50 pounds
(E) 65 pounds

425. The x-ray shown below, which was taken in the plane of the pelvic inlet, demonstrates which of the following types of pelvic morphology?

(A) Anthropoid
(B) Android
(C) Gynecoid
(D) Platypelloid
(E) Trianguloid

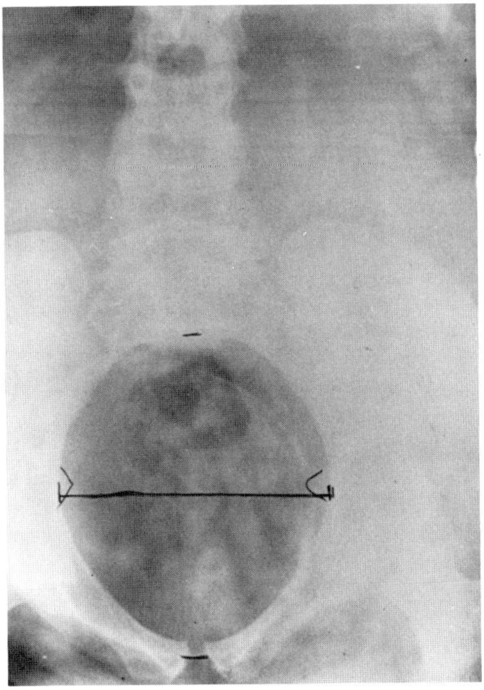

DIRECTIONS: Each question below contains four suggested answers of which **one** or **more** is correct. Choose the answer:

A	if	**1, 2, and 3**	are correct
B	if	**1 and 3**	are correct
C	if	**2 and 4**	are correct
D	if	**4**	is correct
E	if	**1, 2, 3, and 4**	are correct

426. Analysis of amniotic fluid can be useful in diagnosing which of the following disorders?

(1) Fetal hemolytic anemia
(2) Spina bifida
(3) Post-maturity syndrome
(4) Cleft palate

427. Birth of twins is associated with an increased incidence of

(1) prolapsed cord
(2) pre-eclampsia
(3) velementous cord insertion
(4) hydramnios

428. Which of the following statements about the twin-twin transfusion syndrome are true?

(1) The donor twin develops hydramnios more often than the recipient twin
(2) Gross differences may be observed between donor and recipient placentas
(3) The donor twin usually suffers from a hemolytic anemia
(4) The recipient twin can develop widespread thromboses

429. The twin-twin transfusion syndrome can be associated with which of the following?

(1) Diamniotic, monochorionic placentas
(2) Twins of opposite sex
(3) Monoamniotic, monochorionic placentas
(4) Fused diamniotic, dichorionic placentas

430. Which of the following thyroxine-related changes can occur during pregnancy?

(1) Increase of total serum thyroxine
(2) Increase of free thyroxine
(3) Increase of thyroxine-binding globulin
(4) Decrease of thyroid-stimulating hormone

431. Which of the following statements about hypothyroidism are true?

(1) It is uncommon during pregnancy
(2) It is associated with an increased abortion rate
(3) It is associated with an increased stillbirth rate
(4) It is generally improved by pregnancy

432. Which of the following statements about hyperthyroidism in pregnancy are true?

(1) It may cause neonatal thyrotoxicosis
(2) It is harder to control than in a nonpregnant woman
(3) Affected women may be treated with thiourea compounds
(4) It is an indication for interrupting a pregnancy

433. Nausea and vomiting are common in pregnancy. Hyperemesis gravidarum, however, is a much more serious and potentially fatal problem. Findings that should alert the physician to the diagnosis of hyperemesis gravidarum **early** in its course include

(1) electrocardiographic evidence of hypokalemia
(2) weight loss
(3) jaundice
(4) ketonuria

434. In infected women, cytomegalovirus can be recovered from

(1) saliva
(2) cervical secretions
(3) urine
(4) liver biopsy specimens

435. Which of the following hepatic lesions are associated with toxemia of pregnancy?

(1) Periportal hemorrhages
(2) Ischemic lesions
(3) Large subcapsular hematomas
(4) Primary fibrin deposits in hepatic arterioles

436. Which of the following statements about toxemia of pregnancy are true?

(1) The incidence varies widely around the world
(2) Ten percent of women who have had toxemia of pregnancy once will develop it again in a later pregnancy
(3) Elevations in systolic or diastolic blood pressures may be diagnostically significant even at blood pressure values less than 140/90 mm Hg
(4) Young primiparous women have the lowest incidence

437. Maternal hyperparathyroidism can be characterized by which of the following statements?

(1) Diagnosis is made more often after pregnancy than during pregnancy
(2) Neonatal tetany may result
(3) Incidence of pathologic fractures is increased
(4) Fertility, labor, and delivery are adversely affected

438. Which of the following statements about hypoparathyroidism in pregnancy are true?

(1) Its etiology is most commonly iatrogenic
(2) It is best treated with oral calcium and vitamin D
(3) It is a contraindication to breast-feeding
(4) It is associated with a marked increase in spontaneous abortions

SUMMARY OF DIRECTIONS

A	B	C	D	E
1, 2, 3 only	1, 3 only	2, 4 only	4 only	All are correct

439. Which of the following physiologic changes can occur during a normal pregnancy?

(1) Decrease in fasting blood beta-hydroxybutyric acid
(2) Increase in postprandial blood sugar
(3) Increase in fasting blood sugar
(4) Increase in postprandial insulin

440. Pregnancy can be considered diabetogenic because

(1) elevated progesterone levels cause decreased insulin secretion
(2) elevated estrogen levels cause decreased insulin secretion
(3) elevated levels of growth hormone cause decreased insulin secretion
(4) elevated levels of human chorionic somatomammotropin inhibit glucose uptake

441. Pregnancy has which of the following effects on a diabetic woman?

(1) Tendency toward ketoacidosis during early pregnancy
(2) Tendency toward hyperglycemia during early pregnancy
(3) Increase in insulin requirement during early pregnancy
(4) Increase in insulin requirement during late pregnancy

442. Situations that increase the risk of morbidity or mortality for the fetus of a diabetic mother include

(1) maternal ketoacidosis
(2) maternal ketonuria in the absence of diabetic ketoacidosis
(3) maternal hyperglycemia
(4) maternal hypoglycemia

443. Maternal diabetes mellitus is associated with which of the following symptoms in the fetus or neonate?

(1) Macrosomia in the fetus
(2) Delayed pulmonic maturity in the fetus
(3) Hypoglycemia in the newborn
(4) Hypocalcemia in the newborn

444. Which of the following statements about a pregnant woman who has phenylketonuria are true?

(1) If her offspring are mentally retarded, they almost certainly have phenylketonuria
(2) A maternal diet low in phenylalanine and instituted by the third trimester can block development of mental retardation in the child
(3) Recommending an abortion is rarely justified
(4) If the maternal diet is unrestricted, the risk of having a mentally retarded child is nearly 100 percent

445. Chorioangiomas can be described by which of the following statements?

(1) They affect more than 5 percent of placentas
(2) They often are associated with anomalous cord insertions
(3) They often are associated with cords containing only two vessels
(4) They are the most common tumors of the placenta

446. Which of the following statements about placental infarcts are true?

(1) They result from thrombosis of the decidual spiral arterioles
(2) They are present in approximately 5 to 20 percent of all third-trimester deliveries
(3) They occur twice as frequently in white women as in black women
(4) They are frequently associated with pre-eclampsia and essential hypertension

447. Systemic lupus erythematosus is associated with which of the following?

(1) High abortion rate
(2) High stillbirth rate
(3) High prematurity rate
(4) Higher-than-normal female-to-male ratio among liveborn siblings

448. Women who have systemic lupus erythematosus should be counseled that

(1) pregnancy is contraindicated, because it very likely will exacerbate the disease
(2) if they are pregnant, they should have a therapeutic abortion to prevent a progression of their symptoms
(3) their disease is likely to inhibit their fertility
(4) their disease is likely to flare up after delivery

449. Which of the following therapeutic measures are appropriate in the treatment of women who have edema of pregnancy?

(1) Salt restriction
(2) Fluid restriction
(3) Diuretics
(4) Bed rest

450. Injection of labeled dehydroepiandrosterone sulfate into a pregnant woman permits assessment of

(1) fetal adrenal function
(2) placental function
(3) maternal ovarian function
(4) uterine blood flow

451. Urinary estriol levels can decrease in women taking

(1) methenamine mandelate (Mandelamine)
(2) ampicillin
(3) large doses of corticosteroids
(4) phenolphthalein cathartics

SUMMARY OF DIRECTIONS

A	B	C	D	E
1, 2, 3 only	1, 3 only	2, 4 only	4 only	All are correct

452. Erythroblastosis fetalis can be caused by maternal incompatibility with which of the following fetal erythrocyte antigens?

(1) Kell
(2) Kidd
(3) Duffy
(4) Lewis

453. Which of the following statements about Rh_0(D) immune globulin (RhoGAM) are true?

(1) Administration is therapeutically unsuccessful in approximately 1.5 percent of cases
(2) It should never be administered during pregnancy
(3) It usually is given in a dose of 300 μg within 72 hours of delivery of an Rh-positive infant to an unsensitized Rh-negative woman
(4) It can prevent ABO incompatibility

454. A 29-year-old Rh-negative woman, gravida 5, para 4, is 18 weeks pregnant. Her last child had erythroblastosis fetalis and required four exchange transfusions at birth. The father of her current pregnancy is not the father of her other children. Although he is Rh-positive, he is a heterozygote. Which of the following statements are true?

(1) The woman has a 75 percent chance of having an erythroblastotic baby with this pregnancy
(2) The woman should be followed with serum titers, and amniocentesis should be performed when the titers are two dilutions greater than baseline values
(3) If fetal hydrops is demonstrated ultrasonographically or amniographically, intrauterine transfusions should be performed prior to 20 weeks gestation
(4) If intrauterine transfusion is necessary, O-negative blood that has been cross-matched against the mother's serum should be used

455. Which of the following statements describe a direct Coombs' test?

(1) It can be useful in analyzing the cord blood of babies at risk for Rh disease
(2) It involves an antiglobulin reagent made by immunizing rabbits to human immunoglobulin
(3) It cannot be used to quantify the amount of an antibody present
(4) It can be performed on the sera of pregnant Rh-negative women to determine the degree of their Rh sensitization

456. Pregnancy should be strongly discouraged in women who have which of the following?

(1) Atrial septal defect
(2) Ventricular septal defect
(3) Patent ductus arteriosus
(4) Eisenmenger's syndrome

457. Which of the following statements about the lecithin-to-sphingomyelin ratio are true?

(1) It can reflect total muscle mass of the fetus
(2) It rises later than normal if toxemia of pregnancy has developed
(3) It rises earlier than normal if erythroblastosis fetalis has developed
(4) It can reflect fetal surfactant production

458. Signs of fetal postmaturity that may be noted prior to delivery include

(1) oligohydramnios
(2) maternal edema
(3) meconium-stained amniotic fluid
(4) maternal weight loss

459. Which of the following diseases have a positive correlation between maternal infection during pregnancy and congenital anomalies in the fetus?

(1) Rubella
(2) Mumps
(3) Cytomegalovirus
(4) Influenza

460. Maternal infection near term by which of the following viruses can cause severe fetal or neonatal infection?

(1) Group B coxsackievirus
(2) Rubella virus
(3) Chickenpox virus
(4) Herpesvirus hominis, type 2

461. Acute obstruction of the umbilical circulation has been found experimentally to provoke which of the following responses?

(1) A rapid fall in fetal central venous pressure
(2) An almost immediate fall in fetal heart rate
(3) A rapidly mediated humoral effect on the fetal heart
(4) A rapidly mediated response by the fetal heart that can be affected by cutting the vagi

462. Substances that cross the placenta poorly or not at all include

(1) thyroxine
(2) long-acting thyroid stimulator
(3) thyroid-stimulating hormone
(4) propylthiouracil

DIRECTIONS: The groups of questions below consist of lettered choices followed by several numbered items. For each numbered item select the **one** lettered choice with which it is **most** closely associated. Each lettered choice may be used once, more than once, or not at all.

Questions 463-465

For each patient described, choose the diagnostic category (according to the Priscilla White classification) that is most appropriate.

(A) Normal
(B) Class A diabetic
(C) Class B diabetic
(D) Class C diabetic
(E) Class D diabetic

463. The patient is a 17-year-old primigravid woman who was diagnosed as being diabetic at age 9 and is currently taking 30 units of Lente insulin every morning. She is 18 weeks pregnant

464. The patient is a 26-year-old woman, gravida 3, para 2. Her first baby weighed 3.9 kg (8.6 pounds) and her second baby weighed 4.1 kg (9 pounds). A glucose tolerance test is done at 28 weeks gestation after 2 days of carbohydrate loading; the test dose is 100 g of oral glucose. Blood sugars (mg/100 ml) are measured as follows: fasting, 88; 1-hour, 179; 2-hour, 144; 3-hour, 123

465. The patient is a 22-year-old primigravid woman who has a strong family history of diabetes. About six months before becoming pregnant, she had a glucose tolerance test. Although test results were abnormal, she was told that the results indicated chemical diabetes only and that no treatment was necessary. She has never been in ketoacidosis and has no symptoms now. An oral glucose tolerance test given at 28 weeks gestation (same method as described in question 464) reveals the following levels (mg/100 ml): fasting value, 92; 1-hour, 170; 2-hour, 148; 3-hour, 127

Questions 466-472

For each condition that follows, select the study that would be helpful in detecting that condition in utero.

(A) Fetal chromosome count
(B) Fetal sex determination
(C) Amniotic fluid level of alpha-fetoprotein
(D) Enzyme analysis of cultured amniotic fluid cells
(E) None of the above

466. Meningomyelocele

467. Achondroplasia

468. Tay-Sachs disease

469. Turner's syndrome

470. Hurler syndrome

471. Down's syndrome (translocation)

472. Hydrocephaly (without associated spinal cord defects)

Perinatology
General Considerations

Answers

396. The answer is D. *(Villee, p 193.)* The major problem associated with elective cesarean sections is the development in a premature infant of the respiratory distress syndrome. Pulmonic maturation may be delayed in infants of mothers who have chemical or adult-onset diabetes. Although femoral epiphyseal studies and measurement of the biparietal diameter might confirm the dates, only the lecithin-sphingomyelin ratio can give some assurance of pulmonic maturity. The maternal fasting blood sugar level, though it may reflect the development of neonatal hypoglycemia, is not as crucial in the clinical situation of this question as the lecithin-sphingomyelin ratio.

397. The answer is D. *(Ratnoff, p 175.)* Retention of a dead fetus can be associated with the slow release of thromboplastic material into the peripheral circulation. Amniotic fluid embolism, on the other hand, causes a dramatic and rapid intravascular coagulopathy. Disseminated intravascular coagulation caused by sepsis probably results from the exposure of subendothelial collagen to circulating blood. Severe pre-eclampsia can be associated with markedly depressed platelet counts as well as diffuse fibrin deposition in multiple small vessels. Although saline abortions have been implicated in causing disseminated intravascular coagulation, prostaglandin $F_{2\alpha}$ abortions thus far have not.

398. The answer is C. *(Pritchard, ed 15. p 731.)* Rupture of a classic cesarean section scar is several times more likely than rupture of a scar of the lower uterine segment. Because one-third of ruptures of a classic scar occur before the onset of labor (sometimes as much as several weeks before term), cesarean section delivery cannot prevent such ruptures from happening. Rupture of a classic scar is associated with a perinatal mortality rate of at least 50 percent; the maternal mortality rate, however, is most likely no higher than 5 percent.

399. The answer is B. *(Pritchard, ed 15. pp 416-421.)* The initial hemorrhage in placenta previa is usually painless and rarely fatal. If a fetus is premature and if hemorrhaging is not severe, vaginal examination of a woman suspected of having placenta previa frequently can be delayed until 37 weeks of gestation; this delay in the potentially hazardous examination reduces the risk of prematurity, which often is associated with placenta previa. Vaginal examination, when needed to determine whether a low-lying placenta is covering the internal os of the cervix, should be performed in an operating room fully prepared for an emergency cesarean section (i.e., a "double set-up"). Increasing maternal age and multiparity are associated with a higher incidence of placenta previa.

400. The answer is A. *(Pritchard, ed 15. pp 457-458.)* Injection of a radiopaque substance into the uterine cavity produces a characteristic x-ray picture in a woman who has a hydatidiform mole. The individual hydropic villi are outlined by the dye and their grapelike appearance is easily appreciated. Unless an intrauterine pregnancy also is present, no fetal skeleton should be observed in an x-ray of a woman who has a hydatidiform mole.

401. The answer is A. *(Aladjem, pp 5-6.)* During pregnancy, plasma volume increases by about 40 percent and red cell volume increases by about 25 percent. These changes result in a reduction of the packed cell volume and are responsible for the "physiologic anemia" of pregnancy.

402. The answer is C. *(Aladjem, pp 7-8.)* Clinical studies have indicated that although systolic blood pressure remains relatively unchanged throughout pregnancy, diastolic blood pressure decreases significantly by the second trimester. A reduction in peripheral vascular resistance, which is noted following the fourteenth week of pregnancy, is responsible for the change in diastolic pressure; this reduction is caused mainly by the increasing percentage of the cardiac output that passes through the uteroplacental circulation.

403. The answer is E. *(Aladjem, p 23.)* Controlled studies have shown that, during pregnancy, creatinine clearance can vary by ±50 percent when compared to inulin clearance, the accepted measure of glomerular filtration rate. A higher level of plasma creatinine results in tubular excretion; as a consequence, clearance by the kidney appears to be elevated. Creatinine clearance gives an accurate estimate of glomerular filtration rate only when the latter is less than 20 ml/min.

404. The answer is C. *(Burrow, pp 578-579.)* The mother described in the question would be said to have inactive, not previously treated tuberculosis. The chance of reactivation of the disease is 1 to 4.5 percent a year. Isoniazid (INH) should be used preventively in the mother and continued for a year. If the mother has inactive disease that has been treated, the baby need not be treated. If the mother has inactive disease and is currently being treated, it normally would be permissible for her to have contact with the baby, who again need not be treated. However, the patient described presents a special problem. Because she has given evidence of being unreliable, her ability to take INH at the prescribed dosage for the prescribed time is suspect. Placing the baby on preventive INH therapy can endanger the child, if the mother fails to administer the drug faithfully. Thus, the safest course would be to vaccinate the baby with BCG vaccine.

405. The answer is C. *(Burrow, pp 68-69.)* Cerebral hemorrhage is the most common cause of death in women who have eclampsia. Sixty percent of women who die two days or less after the onset of convulsions are found subsequently to have cerebral hemorrhages. Evidence suggests that the pathophysiology of the lesions involves cerebral vasoconstriction.

406. The answer is C. *(Ingemarsson, Am J Obstet Gynecol 125 [1976]: 520.)* Beta-stimulating drugs have been used successfully to inhibit uterine activity. Drugs of this type, such as fenoterol, ritodrine, salbutamol, and terbutaline, stimulate β_2 receptors of the uterus; cardiac β_1 receptors are also stimulated, but only to a minor degree. Propranolol is a beta-blocking agent.

407. The answer is A. *(Burrow, p 421.)* The first response to a primary infection of rubella and other viruses is the elaboration of immunoglobulin M (IgM). Although IgM, once produced, is present for at least several weeks, rising levels of immunoglobulin G (IgG) account for the fact that IgG eventually comprises nearly all antibody detected in the serum. Complement-fixation antibodies usually appear seven to ten days after appearance of the rubella rash.

408. The answer is A. *(Pritchard, ed 15. p 691.)* The three criteria for an x-ray diagnosis of hydrocephaly in utero are a small face in relation to a large head, a hydrocephalic head that is usually globular instead of ovoid, and an often scarcely visible or very thin shadow of a hydrocephalic cranium. In the x-ray shown, the tremendous disproportion between head and body leaves little doubt as to the diagnosis of hydrocephaly.

409. The answer is D. *(Burrow, pp 420, 423.)* A titer of 1:8 obtained by a hemagglutination inhibition (HAI) test may or may not indicate prior exposure to rubella virus. This titer in an exposed patient could represent a false positive result caused by the presence of nonspecific hemagglutinin inhibitors, which can be found in all human sera. On the other hand, a patient who has a titer of 1:8 eighteen days after exposure to rubella could be susceptible and harboring an inapparent infection that has just begun to stimulate manufacture of antibody. If a titer repeated 10 to 14 days later is the same as the first one, the patient is assumed to be immune. If, on the other hand, the repeat titer is 1:32 or greater, the initial titer most likely represented early antibody response to an inapparent infection. Rubella vaccination is contraindicated in pregnant women.

410. The answer is C. *(Burrow, pp 898-899.)* Chronic alcohol abuse, which can cause liver disease, folate deficiency, and many other disorders in a pregnant woman, also can lead to the development of congenital abnormalities in the baby. The chief abnormalities associated with the "fetal alcohol syndrome" are microcephaly, growth retardation, and cardiac anomalies. Chronic abuse of alcohol also may be associated with an increased incidence of mental retardation in the children of affected women.

411. The answer is B. *(Burrow, pp 820-821.)* Achondroplasia is associated with an autosomal dominant pattern of inheritance. However, mutation accounts for 80 percent of all cases of the disorder. Affected women almost always require cesarean section because of the distorted shape of their pelves. Women who have achondroplasia and receive adequate treatment for its associated complications generally have a normal life expectancy.

412. The answer is C. *(Burrow, p 901. Butler Br Med J 2 [1972]: 127-130. Department of Health, Education and Welfare, pp 103-149.)* The incidence of toxemia of pregnancy seems to be decreased in women who smoke during pregnancy; this curious fact, which has yet to be explained, is supported by a number of epidemiologic studies. Offspring of women who smoke more than five cigarettes daily from about the fourth month of pregnancy show decreases in birth weight of as much as 400 g when compared to matched controls. The incidence of premature deliveries, however, has not been found to increase in women who smoke during pregnancy.

413. The answer is B. *(Aladjem, pp 258-260.)* Planimetric studies have demonstrated that the surface area of a normal placenta at term is 11 to 14 square meters. In diseases such as Rh incompatibility, however, placental edema causes marked discrepancies between surface area and total capillary area. Decreased total placental area frequently is associated with placental insufficiency. Because planimetric measurements can only be made in the postpartum state, they are of little diagnostic use.

414. The answer is E. *(Aladjem, p 269. Burrow, p 912.)* The fetal, placental, and maternal compartments have very different enzymatic capacities. Conversion of C-21 to C-19 compounds can occur in the ovaries and the fetal adrenal glands, but not in the placenta. Fetal adrenals convert progesterone to dehydroepiandrosterone, to which a sulfate radical is added by the fetal liver. The placenta has the capacity to convert dehydroepiandrosterone sulfate to estrogens far more efficiently than the maternal compartment.

415. The answer is B. *(Aladjem, pp 268-270.)* Total urinary estrogens at term are markedly elevated when compared to those of a nonpregnant woman. Estriol comprises 80 to 85 percent of this urinary estrogen; its precursors are derived from the fetal liver and adrenal glands. When placental sulfatase activity is diminished, urinary excretion of estriol markedly decreases.

416. The answer is A. *(Burrow, p 417.)* Both viremia and the excretion of virus from the throats of individuals infected with rubella occur five to seven days before the appearance of the characteristic maculopapular rash. The importance of this relationship is that by the time a pregnant woman first notes the appearance of a rash on one of her children, she already has been exposed to the disease and may, in fact, be infected. If one member of a family develops rubella, all other members who are susceptible to the disease usually become infected.

417. The answer is C. *(Adamsons, Am J Obstet Gynecol 96 [1966]: 437.)* Because of its large molecular size and strong electronegativity, heparin cannot cross tissue boundaries easily. Warfarin (Coumadin), on the other hand, easily crosses the placental barrier and thus can cause anticoagulation in a fetus. All of the other drugs listed in the question easily cross the placenta and can be recovered from fetal blood.

418. The answer B. *(Beck, p 454. Ratnoff, p 175.)* Fibrinogen concentrate is obtained from pooled plasma. Compared to a unit of whole blood, it is approximately 30 times more likely to cause hepatitis. Fibrinogen delivered in whole blood, cryoprecipitate, or fresh frozen plasma carries much less risk of hepatitis. Women who have disseminated intravascular coagulation following a placental abruption are more in need of fibrinogen than platelets. Primary fibrinolysis is almost never a contributing factor to the coagulopathies of these women.

419. The answer is C. *(Pritchard, ed 15. pp 148-149.)* The biparietal diameter is figured from the inner table of one area of the fetal skull (one echo) to the outer table of the other. In the echogram shown, the falx is easily seen in the midline. Therefore, line C represents the true biparietal diameter. Line A represents a diagonal from one table of the skull to another. Line B measures the longitudinal length of the skull. Line D represents the distance between the falx and the outer table of the fetal skull, and line E is a chord describing a portion of the circumference. The measurement of the biparietal diameter is essential to modern-day obstetricians because it can establish intrauterine gestational age.

420. The answer is B. *(Aladjem, p 305.)* Deceleration of the fetal heart rate is related to hypoxia. Although fetal hypoxia also leads to a metabolic acidosis, which is reflected by a low arterial pH and increased base deficits, deceleration of the fetal heart rate occurs before development of the acidosis.

421. The answer is C. *(Hon, p 102.)* Late deceleration patterns on a fetal monitoring strip result from fetal hypoxia caused by decreased perfusion, during contractions, of the intervillous spaces. A healthy fetus can tolerate the transient hypoxia resulting from contractions without exhibiting heart rate changes. Thus, late deceleration patterns are ominous, because they indicate that a fetus has very little reserve. Permanent damage of the central nervous system can result if the hypoxia is allowed to persist.

422. The answer is A. *(McCrann, Clin Perinatol 1 [1974]: 242.)* The fetal monitoring strip shown illustrates a uteroplacental insufficiency pattern. In this pattern, deceleration of the heart rate begins after the onset of the contraction, and the lowest rate occurs after the contraction has peaked. In addition there is a very slow return to the baseline. This is an ominous pattern and implies significant fetal hypoxia. Scalp pH sampling is warranted in this situation; and if acidosis is present and the pattern persists with subsequent contractions, rapid delivery should be performed.

423. The answer is D. *(Burrow, pp 110-115.)* Nearly all of the circulatory changes that normally accompany pregnancy are harmful to a woman who has mitral stenosis. Left atrial pressure rises because of increased cardiac output and shortened diastolic filling time; as a result, pulmonary flow is accentuated. Atrial fibrillation may occur suddenly during pregnancy, and pulmonary edema may supervene. Cardioversion may be necessary to reverse atrial fibrillation. Mitral regurgitation is unlikely to be worsened by pregnancy, although prophylaxis for subacute bacterial endocarditis is indicated for such women. Aortic stenosis is unusual as a pure lesion; problems, if they are going to develop at all, are most likely to develop in the immediate postpartum period, when rapid volume shifts can occur. Aortic regurgitation also is rare as a pure lesion and again is most likely to cause problems just after delivery.

424. The answer is D. *(Aladjem, p 294.)* Traction forces applied to the head during a forceps delivery should not exceed 50 pounds. The safe upper limit for compression forces, however, is only 4 to 5 pounds. Forces in excess of these may be associated with fetal trauma.

425. The answer is A. *(Pritchard, ed 15. pp 231-232.)* The anteroposterior diameter of the inlet of the anthropoid pelvis shown in the x-ray is greater than the transverse diameter. The anterior segment of an anthropoid pelvis is narrow, the ischial spines often are prominent, and the side walls may be somewhat convergent. In one American study, the anthropoid pelvis was found to be nearly twice as common (40 percent to 23 percent) in nonwhite women as in white women. This type of pelvis is far more likely than a gynecoid pelvis to be a source of dystocia.

426. The answer is A (1, 2, 3). *(Burrow, pp 918-923.)* Because spectrophotometric analysis of amniotic fluid can determine the concentration of indirect bilirubin, which is a reflection of fetal red cell hemolysis, the procedure is a mainstay in the management of patients who have Rh incompatibility. If meconium is present in amniotic fluid aspirated from a pregnant woman who is at least two weeks past her due date, the presence of post-maturity syndrome must be assumed until proven otherwise. Open neural tube defects, such as spina bifida, can be diagnosed by the high levels of alpha-fetoprotein in the amniotic fluid; closed neural tube defects, on the other hand, are not accompanied by increased concentrations of this substance. Cleft palate cannot be diagnosed at this time by chromosomal or biochemical analyses of amniotic fluid.

427. The answer is E (all). *(Benirschke, NY State J Med 61 [1961]: 4499. Robertson, Obstet Gynecol 23 [1964]: 330.)* In one series of 450 twins, the incidence of cord prolapse was 3 percent for the first twin and 5 percent for the second; the overall hospital incidence was 1 percent during the same period of time. In the same series the incidence of pre-eclampsia in mothers of twins was reported to be 32 percent. Twins also have a greatly increased incidence of velementous cord insertion and therefore are at risk for rupturing a vasa praevia. Hydramnios has been reported to occur in 12.5 percent of twins.

428. The answer is C (2, 4). *(Benirschke, NY State J Med 61 [1961]: 4499.)* In the twin-twin transfusion syndrome, the donor twin is always anemic, due not to a hemolytic process but to the direct transfer of blood to the recipient twin. The recipient may suffer thromboses secondary to hypertransfusion and subsequent hemoconcentration. Although the donor placenta is usually pale and somewhat atrophied, that of the recipient is congested and enlarged. Hydramnios can develop in either twin but, because of circulatory overload, is more frequent in the recipient. Hydramnios when it occurs in the donor is due to congestive heart failure caused by severe anemia.

429. The answer is B (1, 3). *(Benirschke, NY State J Med 61 [1961]: 4499.)* The twin-twin transfusion syndrome is a result of vascular anastomoses between the arterial circulation of one twin and the venous circulation of the other. Because a monochorionic placenta must be present, dizygotic twins are not affected by the twin-twin transfusion syndrome, even if their placentas are fused.

430. The answer is B (1, 3). *(Burrow, pp 196-201.)* Probably because of increased estrogen levels, pregnancy is associated with an increase in the amounts of many proteins in the serum, among them thyroxine-binding globulin. In order to maintain normal levels of free thyroxine and triiodothyronine, more total thyroxine must be produced to tie up some of the excess binding sites on the carrier protein. Therefore, the total serum thyroxine concentration increases while the level of free thyroxine stays constant. Thyroid-stimulating hormone (TSH) levels are slightly increased during early pregnancy but by term are back in the normal range, as measured by radioimmunoassay. There are some data to suggest that TSH-like activity also is increased in pregnancy, possibly due to a placental factor, either human chorionic gonadotropin or human chorionic thyrotropin. This explanation seems to apply especially to molar pregnancies.

431. The answer is A (1, 2, 3). *(Burrow, pp 213-216.)* Why hypothyroidism is uncommon during pregnancy is not known. The most widely supported explanation is that many hypothyroid patients are anovulatory and thus do not easily become pregnant. However, if a hypothyroid patient does become pregnant, her disease, if untreated, could lead to abortion and stillbirth. For this reason, most perinatologists prefer to treat hypothyroidism vigorously during pregnancy. For example, if a woman who has been placed on low-dose thyroid replacement for poorly documented hypothyroidism becomes pregnant, administration of thyroid hormone probably should be increased to full replacement dose for the remainder of the pregnancy; after delivery, hormone therapy should be discontinued in order to re-evaluate thyroid function.

432. The answer is B (1, 3). *(Burrow, pp 226-236.)* Hyperthyroidism in pregnancy may cause neonatal thyrotoxicosis. The mechanism is not the transmission of triiodothyronine or thyroxine to the baby but rather the crossing of long-acting thyroid stimulator (LATS) to the baby with subsequent hyperfunction of the fetal thyroid gland. Not all hyperthyroid women have LATS; and it is only those who do who are at risk for neonatal thyrotoxicosis. The usual treatment for hyperthyroidism in pregnancy is administration of thiourea compounds, although in some centers surgery is popular. Hyperthyroidism often becomes less severe during pregnancy, especially during the last trimester, at which time requirements for thiourea drugs often decrease. Because hyperthyroidism is a treatable disorder, it is not an indication for terminating a pregnancy.

433. The answer is C (2, 4). *(Burrow, pp 285-292.)* Hyperemesis gravidarum is intractable vomiting of pregnancy and is associated with disturbed nutrition. Early signs of the disorder include weight loss, up to 5 percent of body weight, and acetonuria. Because vomiting causes potassium loss, electrocardiographic evidence of potassium depletion, such as inverted T waves and prolonged Q-T and P-R intervals, is usually a later finding. Jaundice also is a later finding and is probably due to fatty infiltration of the liver; occasionally acute hepatic necrosis occurs. Hypokalemic nephropathy with isosthenuria may occur late. Hypoproteinemia also may result, caused by poor diet as well as by albuminuria. Patients who have hyperemesis gravidarum are best treated (if the disease is early in its course) with parenteral fluids and electrolytes, sedation, rest, vitamins, and antiemetics if necessary. In some cases, isolation of the patient is necessary. Very slow reinstitution of oral feeding is permitted after dehydration and electrolyte disturbances are corrected. Therapeutic abortion may be necessary in rare instances; usually, however, the disease tends to improve as pregnancy progresses.

434. The answer is E (all). *(Burrow, p 426.)* Cytomegalovirus can be recovered from the urine, saliva, or cervical secretions of infected women; the virus also can be found in specimens from a liver biopsy. Urine is the best source for recovering cytomegalovirus, which may be present in concentrations as high as 1 million virus particles per milliliter. Cultures of the virus, which is slow-growing, may not be positive until a month or more has passed.

435. The answer is A (1, 2, 3). *(Burrow, p 68.)* Toxemia of pregnancy is associated with two types of hepatic lesions: periportal hemorrhages, which eventually are supplanted by fibrin deposits, and ischemic lesions, which can vary greatly in size and severity. It has been hypothesized that it is the spasm of hepatic arterioles, and not the primary deposition of fibrin, that is responsible for the hemorrhagic lesions.

436. The answer is B (1, 3). *(Burrow, pp 75-76.)* Worldwide, the incidence of toxemia varies from a low of 2 percent in the Far East to almost 30 percent in Puerto Rico. Peak incidences occur in two groups: young primiparous women and multiparous women who are older than 35 years of age. Moreover, women who have had toxemia of pregnancy in the past have a 33 percent chance of developing the disease again in later pregnancies. Because of the difficulty in defining "normal" blood pressures for pregnant women, elevations in the systolic component (of 20 mm Hg or more) or the diastolic component (of 10 mm Hg or more) during pregnancy are defined as "abnormal," notwithstanding the absolute blood pressure values.

437. The answer is A (1, 2, 3). *(Burrow, pp 265-268.)* Hyperparathyroidism, which often is caused by a parathyroid adenoma, is characterized by elevated levels of serum calcium and symptoms associated with hypercalcemia. These symptoms include weakness, nausea, polyuria, and polydipsia; renal stones and pathologic fractures also can occur. Because the milder of these symptoms may be seen in normal pregnancies, the presence of hyperparathyroidism may be missed during pregnancy. More than half of the babies born to hyperparathyroid mothers have neonatal tetany, a first clue, in many instances, in diagnosing the disease in the mother. The tetany is due to hypocalcemia in the newborn and occurs usually at 5 to 14 days of age. Hyperparathyroid patients do not have increased infertility problems, and labor and delivery appear to be normal, although there is some evidence that the incidence of small-for-dates babies is increased.

438. The answer is A (1, 2, 3). *(Burrow, pp 268-271.)* Hypoparathyroidism is most commonly iatrogenic, occurring when the parathyroid glands have been inadvertently removed at the time of thyroidectomy. The disease is characterized by low levels of serum calcium and high levels of serum phosphate. The usual treatment is oral calcium and vitamin D. Hypoparathyroid mothers should not breast-feed their children, because the calcium drain of breast-feeding may worsen their hypocalcemia. The outcome of pregnancy in the hypoparathyroid patient who is under treatment should be excellent. If tetany occurs during pregnancy, hypoparathyroidism should be suspected, especially if the patient has had previous thyroid surgery; the most common cause of tetany during pregnancy, however, is alkalosis.

439. The answer is C (2, 4). *(Burrow, pp 175-179.)* During pregnancy fasting blood glucose levels generally decrease, probably because the fetus, needing tremendous amounts of glucose, takes glucose at the expense of the mother. In addition, the maternal response to fasting is accentuated by pregnancy and results in exaggerated starvation ketosis and increased fasting levels of beta-hydroxybutyric acid (a ketone body). For a number of reasons, insulin is less effective during pregnancy in diminishing blood glucose. Postprandial blood glucose therefore tends to be higher than in the nonpregnant state, and results of a glucose tolerance test must be interpreted differently. To offset anti-insulin effects, insulin production is augmented during the normal pregnancy, and postprandial insulin levels are increased.

440. The answer is D (4). *(Burrow, pp 174-175.)* The tendency for pregnancy to be diabetogenic is thought to be due mainly to the anti-insulin effects of many of the hormones secreted by the placenta as well as to the possible effect of insulin receptors on the placenta itself. Human chorionic somatomammotropin (also known as human placental lactogen) is present in huge amounts in the maternal circulation during the third trimester. Its lipolytic and other actions inhibit glucose uptake and manufacture and therefore stimulate insulin production to rise. Levels of pituitary growth hormone are decreased, especially during late pregnancy, and probably have little to do with increased insulin needs. Estrogen and probably progesterone, both of which are present in increased amounts during pregnancy, probably act as peripheral insulin antagonists and therefore would not lead to decreased insulin secretion.

441. The answer is D (4). *(Burrow, pp 179-180.)* Although during early pregnancy the diabetogenic effects of placental hormones are not marked, there is still a net transfer of glucose from mother to fetus. For this reason, there is a tendency toward maternal hypoglycemia rather than hyperglycemia; ketoacidosis is rare and insulin reactions are common. In fact, one of the first symptoms of pregnancy in a diabetic woman may be hypoglycemia and decreasing insulin need. Later on in pregnancy, however, insulin requirements increase markedly and are about two-thirds higher than before pregnancy. Hypoglycemia now becomes less of a problem than ketoacidosis.

442. The answer is A (1, 2, 3). *(Burrow, pp 173, 181-186.)* Sophisticated management of high-risk diabetic individuals has reduced the incidence of diabetic ketoacidosis. When it occurs in pregnant women, however, it is associated with an extremely high fetal mortality rate. In addition, ketonuria in the absence of acidosis (i.e., starvation ketosis) has been correlated with decreased intelligence quotients in the offspring. Perinatal mortality has been correlated to hyperglycemia even in the absence of ketoacidosis, and this finding is the cornerstone of current recommendations urging strict control of diabetes during pregnancy. A correlation between maternal hypoglycemia and fetal morbidity or mortality has not been shown; in fact, rather severe episodes of hypoglycemia have been reported to have no effect on the outcome of pregnancy.

443. The answer is E (all). *(Burrow, pp 182-184.)* Maternal diabetes, especially of the milder classes, is associated with macrosomia in the fetus. Glucose crosses the placenta freely by facilitated diffusion, but insulin does not. The fetus, in response to the chronic glucose load, secretes increased quantities of insulin. Insulin acts as a growth hormone in the fetus, and the fetus becomes macrosomic. At delivery, the fetus is removed from the relatively glucose-rich maternal environment but continues to secrete increased amounts of insulin. Thus, the fetus may become hypoglycemic in the early hours of life unless early feeding, sometimes even intravenous glucose, is begun. Hypocalcemia may occur in as many as one-fourth of infants of diabetic mothers, possibly as a result of fetal parathyroid suppression stemming from maternal hypercalcemia. Lastly, fetal lung maturity, as measured by the lecithin-to-sphingomyelin ratio, may be delayed, especially in the infants of mothers who have mild diabetes.

444. The answer is D (4). *(Burrow, p 820.)* The chance that a women who has phenylketonuria will have a retarded child is almost 100 percent if her blood levels of phenylalanine are not kept within normal limits. These retarded offspring rarely have the disease themselves. Recent evidence suggests that institution of a low-phenylalanine diet before conception may prevent the development of retardation, if the diet is continued throughout pregnancy. A low-phenylalanine diet begun after conception, however, seems to be of no value in preventing retardation. Because of the high risk of severe mental retardation in affected offspring, interruption of pregnancy has been recommended for women who have phenylketonuria and either have never been placed on low-phenylalanine diets or were started on their diets after becoming pregnant.

445. The answer is D (4). *(Aladjem, p 243.)* Chorioangiomas are the most common placental tumor, occurring in approximately 1 percent of placentas. Despite attempts to correlate the presence of this tumor with hydramnios and fetal anomalies, no significant effect on fetal morbidity and mortality has been demonstrated, unless the size of the tumor is very great.

446. The answer is E (all). *(Aladjem, p 243.)* Although the incidence of placental infarction in the United States is twice as high for white women as it is for black women, the perinatal mortality rate shows just the opposite relationship. Placental infarcts, which are caused by thrombosis of the decidual spiral arterioles, are present in up to 20 percent of all placentas at delivery. Diseases, such as essential hypertension and pre-eclampsia, that can cause the vascular changes associated with placental infarction may be more important in causing fetal compromise than the infarct itself.

447. The answer is E (all). *(Burrow, p 790.)* The incidence of spontaneous abortion is about 40 percent after the clinical onset of systemic lupus erythematosus. If renal disease is present, the abortion rate is higher still. Prematurity has been found to be present in as many as one-third of deliveries, and stillbirths occur with increased frequency. The sex ratio also is changed in the offspring of women who have lupus erythematosus, with a decrease in the ratio of liveborn males to total liveborn siblings. The preponderance of females with lupus may, in fact, be due to the high mortality rate among male siblings antenatally.

448. The answer is D (4). *(Burrow, pp 786-794.)* Studies on the effect of pregnancy on the course of systemic lupus erythematosus have been inconsistent in their findings. Some studies suggest a worsening of the disease, while others show remission or no effect at all. If a woman who is informed that her lupus might get worse during pregnancy still wants to have a child, she may be supported in her plans. In most cases therapeutic abortion is not indicated, because the postpartum flareup, especially in renal disease, may occur whether the pregnancy has been terminated by abortion or delivery. For some very sick patients, however, abortion may be lifesaving. Only in cases involving severe renal disease does lupus seem to decrease the fertility rate.

449. The answer is D (4). *(Burrow, pp 929-930.)* Women who have edema of pregnancy have traditionally been treated with salt restriction and diuretics. It is now clear, however, that sodium and water retention are normal processes during pregnancy. More water than sodium is retained, so unnecessary salt restriction and diuretics may cause intravascular depletion. Diuretics also may cause sodium and potassium depletion in the mother. Thiazide diuretics have been implicated in hemorrhagic pancreatitis and deterioration of glucose tolerance in the mother and in thrombocytopenia in the newborn. The best treatment for edema of pregnancy probably is extra bed rest in the lateral recumbent position, which should improve renal perfusion.

450. The answer is C (2, 4). *(Burrow, p 912.)* Less than 0.2 percent of circulating dehydroepiandrosterone sulfate (DS) is converted to estrogen by nonpregnant women. In late pregnancy, however, the placenta converts from 75 to 80 percent of maternal circulating DS to estrone and estradiol. The clearance rate of labeled DS is felt to reflect uterine blood flow, and the production of labeled estradiol is an indicator of placental function.

451. The answer is E (all). *(Burrow, p 910.)* Methenamine mandelate (Mandelamine), ampicillin, corticosteroids, and phenolphthalein all can reduce urinary estriol levels. Formaldehyde produced by the acid hydrolysis of methenamine mandelate in the urine can degrade estrogens. Hydrolysis of estrogen conjugates is inhibited by phenolphthalein. Large daily doses of cortisol, which can cross the placenta, suppress fetal adrenal function and therefore inhibit production of estriol precursors. Ampicillin use is thought to cause fecal loss of steroids, which results from an inhibition in the gastrointestinal tract of the hydrolysis of biliary estriol conjugates.

452. The answer is A (1, 2, 3). *(Queenan, p 13. Williams, pp 502-503, 1266-1279.)* Erythroblastosis fetalis, also known as isoimmune hemolytic disease of the newborn, results from the transplacental passage of maternal blood-group antibodies and subsequent destructive reaction with fetal erythrocyte antigens. It is theoretically possible for any blood-group antigen with the exceptions of Lewis and I antigens to cause erythroblastosis fetalis. Lewis and I antigens are not present on fetal red blood cells; furthermore, the antibodies to these two antigens are immunoglobulin M, which does not cross the placenta.

453. The answer is B (1, 3). *(Scott, Contemporary Obstet Gynecol 8[1976]: 27.)* Rh_0(D) immune globulin (RhoGAM) is a concentrated sterile solution of human immunoglobulin G that contains anti-Rh_0(D); it can prevent the formation of active Rh_0(D) antibody in women, therefore impeding the development of Rh hemolytic disease of the newborn in subsequent deliveries. Rh_0(D) immune globulin is usually given in an intramuscular dose of 300 μg within 72 hours of delivery. The failure rate, which is reported to be 1 to 2 percent, is attributed either to the development of sensitization in a subsequent pregnancy or to an unrecognized sensitization that already exists when the drug is administered. Rh_0(D) immune globulin is of no benefit in ABO incompatibility.

454. The answer is D (4). *(Queenan, pp 33-55, 152-218.)* An Rh-negative woman married to a heterozygous Rh-positive man has a 50 percent chance of having an Rh-positive baby. Spectrophotometric analyses of the woman's amniotic fluid should be performed to detect bilirubin pigment; they should begin at 22 to 23 weeks gestation and be repeated every two weeks until delivery. (Serum titers are very inaccurate in women who were sensitized in previous pregnancies.) If the level of bilirubin pigment suggests imminent fetal demise, intrauterine transfusion of the pulmonically immature fetus is indicated. Transfusion before 23 to 24 weeks gestation should not be attempted because of technical difficulties and the extremely poor chance of success at so early a stage. When intrauterine transfusions are performed, O-negative blood that is cross-matched against the mother's serum should be used.

455. The answer is A (1, 2, 3). *(Queenan, p 17.)* The direct Coombs' test, which uses human antiglobulin derived from immunized rabbits, is performed on blood cells to determine if they are coated with antibody. A direct Coombs' test, therefore, can be useful in analyzing the cord blood of an infant who is at risk for Rh disease. Quantification of antibody titers can be achieved by doing serial dilutions of the indirect Coombs' test, which analyzes serum.

456. The answer is D (4). *(Burrow, pp 120-127.)* Eisenmenger's syndrome consists of severe pulmonary hypertension combined with a bidirectional or reversed shunt through a patent ductus arteriosus or an atrial or ventricular septal defect. The death rate during pregnancy for women who have this syndrome is higher than in any other form of congenital heart disease. Death usually occurs at or just after delivery and is probably associated with a sudden drop in peripheral vascular resistance. Atrial and ventricular septal defects, in the absence of pulmonary hypertension and right-to-left shunting, rarely cause problems during pregnancy. Unless shunting is minimal, a patent ductus arteriosus is usually detected by the time a woman becomes pregnant. Again, only reversal of the shunt should pose any problems.

457. The answer is D (4). *(Burrow, pp 919-923.)* The lecithin-to-sphingomyelin (L/S) ratio, measured from amniotic-fluid samples, is a barometer of pulmonic maturity. If the L/S ratio is above whatever value denotes maturity in a particular laboratory, respiratory distress syndrome will probably not be present in the newborn. Lecithin seems to be involved in surfactant activity, and its secretion from the lungs into the amniotic fluid yields information about surfactant production in the fetal lungs. Amniotic-fluid creatinine values have been used to document fetal maturity; but because they also can reflect the muscle mass of a fetus, they are not as valid as the L/S ratio. The L/S ratio may reach maturity levels earlier in stressful situations, as in toxemia of pregnancy, for example. Delay in pulmonic maturation occurs in association with mild diabetes but not with erythroblastosis fetalis.

458. The answer is B (1, 3). *(Pritchard, ed 15. pp 797-799.)* Although all infants beyond 42 weeks gestation are considered postmature, the postmaturity syndrome does not affect all these infants. The syndrome itself consists of wasted subcutaneous tissues, peeling skin, long nails, diminished amniotic fluid, and meconium staining of amniotic fluid and baby. Prior to birth, ultrasound examination can detect a decreased amniotic fluid volume, and amniocentesis can be used to determine the presence or absence of meconium. The presence of postmaturity syndrome correlates with an increase in the stillbirth rate and an increase in neonatal complications, the most common of which are meconium aspiration and hypoglycemia. The incidence of cord entanglement also is increased, probably due to diminished amniotic fluid volumes. When gestation is prolonged beyond the forty-second week of pregnancy and meconium or oligohydramnios is present, prompt delivery should be performed.

459. The answer is B (1, 3). *(Burrow, pp 416-433.)* Rubella syndrome in the newborn secondary to rubella infection during pregnancy (especially, but not exclusively, during the first trimester) is well known. Although cytomegalovirus infection is less familiar, it is thought to cause congenital anomalies in about 5,000 newborns every year in the United States. The abnormalities are usually in the central nervous system and include microcephaly, cerebral calcifications, deafness, and other mental and motor disabilities. Although there have been some suggestions that influenza epidemics have led to a subsequent rise in the incidence of childhood leukemia, this relationship has not been established; in fact, there is no proof that influenza is associated with any anomalies. Mumps is relatively common during pregnancy, but prospective studies have failed to show any associated congenital anomalies.

460. The answer is E (all). *(Burrow, pp 416-433, 479.)* A mild Group B coxsackievirus infection of the mother during the antepartum period may give rise to a virulent infection in the newborn, sometimes resulting in a fatal encephalomyocarditis. A maternal rubella infection may cause neonatal hepatosplenomegaly, petechial rash, and jaundice; in addition, viral shedding may last for months or years. Herpes zoster, the causative agent of varicella (chickenpox), is an especially dangerous organism for the newborn. Varicella is rare in pregnancy, but if it occurs shortly before delivery, the viremia may spread to the fetus before protective maternal antibodies have had a chance to form. Congenital varicella can be fatal to the newborn; the increasing availability of zoster immune globulin, however, may allow clinicians to attack the infection before significant fetal viremia has developed. Herpesvirus can be acquired by the fetus as it passes down the genital tract and can cause a severe, often fatal herpes infection in the newborn.

461. The answer is C (2, 4). *(Aladjem, pp 306-307.)* Fetal heart rate has been shown to drop almost immediately when the umbilical circulation has been obstructed in experimental situations. This response is a reflex action that is caused by the sudden rise in central venous pressure and that disappears if the vagi are severed. A more prolonged obstruction of the umbilical circulation can cause a delayed fall in the fetal heart rate secondary to progressive asphyxia.

462. The answer is B (1, 3). *(Burrow, pp 218-219, 226-236.)* Thyroxine crosses the placenta poorly, if at all. For this reason, a hyperthyroid mother does not transmit her hyperthyroidism to the fetus, and giving thyroid hormone to a hypothyroid mother will not raise fetal thyroxine levels significantly. Thyroid-stimulating hormone also does not cross to the fetus. On the other hand, propylthiouracil (PTU), an antithyroid drug, crosses easily and may suppress fetal thyroid function. Hyperthyroid women taking large doses of PTU therefore run the risk of having goitrous babies. Some clinicians, hoping to reverse the effect of PTU on the fetus, have given thyroxine to the mother; theoretically, however, this should not work, because the thyroid hormone should not get to the fetus. Long-acting thyroid stimulator (LATS) is present in many patients who have Graves' disease. Because LATS can cross the placenta, LATS levels should be obtained from such patients, and the pediatrician should be alerted to possible neonatal thyrotoxicosis if LATS is present.

463-465. The answers are: 463-E, 464-A, 465-B. *(Burrow, pp 177-179.)* The Priscilla White classification is the most widely used descriptive categorization of diabetes in pregnant women. To a certain extent, as the classes progress alphabetically, the fetal prognosis becomes increasingly poor. A class A diabetic patient is one who either is diagnosed during pregnancy and needs no insulin or, if diagnosed before pregnancy, was asymptomatic and needed no treatment. A class B diabetic patient is overtly diabetic and was diagnosed after the age of 20; in addition, the duration of the disease is less than 10 years. A class C diabetic woman was diagnosed either between the ages of 10 and 20 years or from 10 to 20 years ago. Diagnosis of a class D diabetic woman was made either before the age of 10 or more than 20 years ago.

The normal values for a glucose tolerance test during pregnancy differ from those of nonpregnant women. With two days of carbohydrate loading and a 100-gram oral glucose tolerance test, a patient, to be considered diabetic, must exceed two of the following four blood-sugar values (mg/100 ml): fasting, 90; 1-hour, 165; 2-hour, 145; 3-hour, 125. If serum or plasma levels are measured, the standards are 14 percent higher.

466-472. The answers are: 466-C, 467-E, 468-D, 469-A, 470-D, 471-E, 472-E. *(Burrow, p 810. Golbus, Obstet Gynecol 48[1976]: 497.)* Aneuploidy can be detected simply by counting fetal chromosomes; the diagnosis of aneuploid disorders, such as Turner's syndrome (45,XO) and trisomy 21 (classic Down's syndrome) can be confirmed by karyotype. Because individuals who have translocation Down's syndrome have 46 chromosomes, a chromosome count would be unrewarding; modern chromosome-banding techniques, however, can demonstrate this abnormality during analysis of the karyotype. Although achondroplasia is an inherited, autosomal dominant disorder, it cannot be detected by karyotypic analysis at this time.

Meningomyelocoele and other open neural-tube defects have markedly elevated amniotic fluid levels of alpha-fetoprotein, probably as a result of the transudation of this protein across the membrane covering the defect. If a neural-tube defect is completely covered with skin, however, the alpha-fetoprotein level may be within normal limits; an example of such closed defects is hydrocephaly that is not associated with spinal cord lesions.

Tay-Sachs disease results from a defect in the synthesis of hexosaminidase A. Hurler syndrome is caused by a deficiency of the enzyme α-L-iduronidase. Both disorders can be detected by enzyme analysis of cultured fetal cells grown from amniotic fluid.

Perinatology
Genetics

Michael T. Mennuti

DIRECTIONS: Each question below contains five suggested answers. Choose the **one best** response to each question.

473. The karyotype below is most likely to be associated with a

(A) normal woman
(B) triple X woman
(C) child who has multiple malformations
(D) spontaneously aborted fetus
(E) none of the above

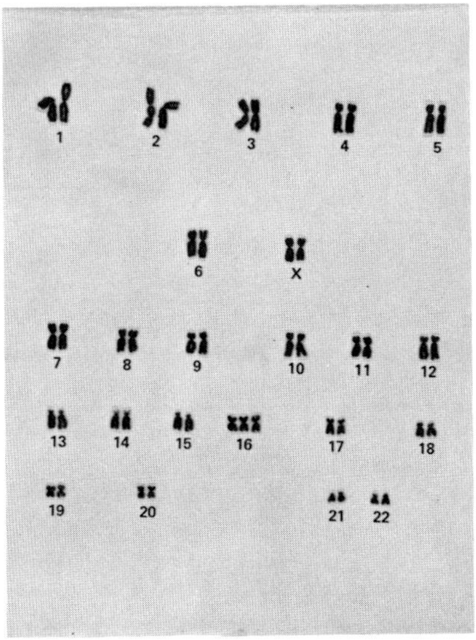

474. What percentage of fetuses who have a 45,XO chromosome constitution are lost prior to birth?

(A) 10 percent
(B) 25 percent
(C) 33 percent
(D) 50 percent
(E) 98 percent

475. A 27-year-old, healthy, pregnant woman and her husband want to know the likelihood of their child being born with cystic fibrosis. The woman had two brothers affected by this disorder who died during childhood. Neither she nor her husband knows of any other family members affected by the disease. Given that the carrier frequency in the population is 1:25, the risk that the child will have cystic fibrosis is

(A) 1:2,500
(B) 1:625
(C) 1:300
(D) 1:150
(E) 1:100

476. The chromosomal abnormality most often detected in first trimester abortuses is

(A) Turner's syndrome
(B) polyploidy
(C) autosomal monosomy
(D) autosomal trisomy
(E) unbalanced translocation

477. The percentage of pregnancy loss that can be attributed to second trimester amniocentesis is

(A) less than 1 percent
(B) 1 to 2 percent
(C) 3 to 4 percent
(D) 5 percent
(E) more than 5 percent

478. The karyotype shown below is most consistent with

(A) Turner's syndrome
(B) Down's syndrome
(C) a translocation carrier
(D) a triple X female
(E) none of the above

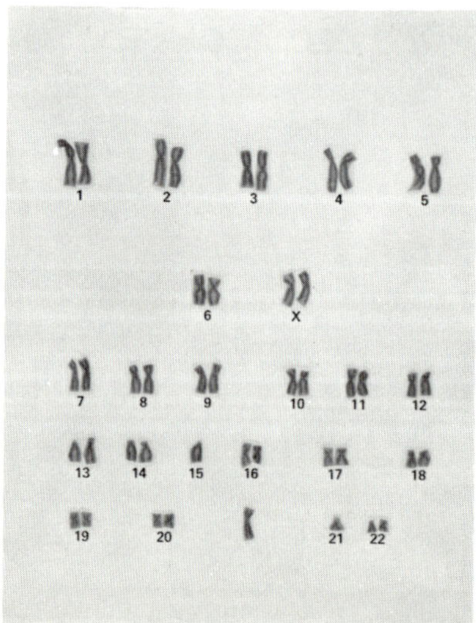

DIRECTIONS: Each question below contains four suggested answers of which **one** or **more** is correct. Choose the answer:

A	if	**1, 2, and 3**	are correct
B	if	**1 and 3**	are correct
C	if	**2 and 4**	are correct
D	if	**4**	is correct
E	if	**1, 2, 3, and 4**	are correct

479. Turner's syndrome can be associated with which of the following karyotypes?

(1) 46,XXr
(2) 46,XXp-
(3) 46,X,i(Xq)
(4) 46,X,i(Xp)

480. The sex of a fetus can be predicted during the second trimester of pregnancy by which of the following techniques?

(1) Karyotyping of cultured amniotic fluid cells
(2) Staining of amniotic fluid cells to demonstrate Y chromosomes
(3) Staining of amniotic fluid cells to demonstrate nuclear sex chromatin (Barr bodies)
(4) Measurement of the amniotic fluid concentration of sex steriods

481. A 23-year-old woman, gravida 2 para 1, wants to know the prenatal diagnosis of her unborn child. Her first child, who was delivered by cesarean section, had anencephaly. An ultrasound examination performed one week ago (at 15 weeks gestation) revealed an anterior placenta and a fetal biparietal diameter consistent with the gestational age as determined by menstrual history. You advise the woman that

(1) an elevated level of alpha-fetoprotein in the amniotic fluid may not necessarily indicate a neural tube defect
(2) an elevated level of alpha-fetoprotein in the amniotic fluid is as likely to indicate a closed neural tube defect as an open neural tube defect
(3) the midtrimester ultrasound examination makes the diagnosis of recurrent anencephaly highly unlikely in this instance
(4) repeated measurement of the concentration of alpha-fetoprotein in maternal serum can substitute for amniocentesis

SUMMARY OF DIRECTIONS

A	B	C	D	E
1, 2, 3 only	1, 3 only	2, 4 only	4 only	All are correct

482. Which of the following statements about X-linked dominant disorders are true?

(1) All daughters of an affected man will be affected
(2) Women are affected more frequently than men
(3) None of the sons of an affected man will be affected
(4) One-half of the sons of an affected woman will be affected

483. Which of the following statements describe gonadal development in women?

(1) Migration of germ cells to the primitive gonad begins in the first trimester of fetal development
(2) Mitotic proliferation of germ cells occurs in the gonad during fetal development
(3) The number of germ cells reaches a peak total of about 6 million
(4) Degeneration (atresia) of germ cells begins at the time of puberty and continues until the menopause

484. Which of the following statements describe a carrier of a balanced 14/21 (D/G) translocation?

(1) Amniocentesis can detect offspring who have translocation Down's syndrome as well as those who are balanced carriers
(2) Karyotype analysis would reveal 45 chromosomes in each cell
(3) Chromosome studies of members of a carrier's family are indicated to detect others who may be at risk for having children with Down's syndrome
(4) The risk for bearing children who have Down's syndrome is the same whether the husband or the wife is the carrier

485. Which of the following statements about a pregnant woman who has phenylketonuria are true?

(1) If the father carries the gene, the risk that the child be be affected is 25 percent
(2) If the father carries the gene, prenatal diagnosis and selective abortion can avert the birth of affected children
(3) In spite of neonatal screening and the institution of low-phenylalanine diets, individuals with phenylketonuria rarely survive to the reproductive years
(4) Children born to mothers who have phenylketonuria have a high frequency of mental retardation

DIRECTIONS: The groups of questions below consist of lettered choices followed by several numbered items. For each numbered item select the **one** lettered choice with which it is **most** closely associated. Each lettered choice may be used once, more than once, or not at all.

Questions 486-490

For each of the following clinical situations, select the most appropriate risk figure.

(A) Equal to that of the U.S. population
(B) 1 percent
(C) 5 percent
(D) 25 percent
(E) None of the above

486. A 21-year-old pregnant woman, whose father had Huntington's chorea and died last year at age 47, wants to know what the chance is that her unborn child will develop the disease. She has been evaluated by a neurologist, who finds no evidence of the disorder in her

487. A Jewish couple of Ashkenazi ancestry, who are considering having a child, request information about the risk that the child will be born with Tay-Sachs disease

488. A 23-year-old woman has a son with Down's syndrome (47,XY,+21). She wishes to know the risk that any subsequent children will have the disorder

489. A 27-year-old pregnant woman wants to know her risk for having a child with Down's syndrome. Her 15-year-old sister (47,XX,+21) has the disorder

490. A 26-year-old woman has had one child with spina bifida. During her second pregnancy, prenatal diagnosis detects an open neural tube defect in the fetus. Following termination of that pregnancy, the woman and her husband request information regarding the risk for this disorder in future pregnancies

Questions 491-495

Match the following.

(A) First meiotic division
(B) Second meiotic division
(C) Both
(D) Neither

491. Results in a reduced number of chromosomes

492. Is arrested during fetal life in the female gonad

493. Is completed during follicular development and ovulation

494. Is subject to errors of nondisjunction resulting in gametes with chromosomal abnormalities

495. Is arrested during fetal life in the male gonad

Questions 496-500

Match the following.

(A) Individuals who have congenital adrenal hyperplasia due to C-17 hydroxylase deficiency
(B) Individuals who have androgen insensitivity due to receptor defect (testicular feminization)
(C) Both
(D) Neither

496. 46,XY chromosome constitution

497. Feminization at puberty

498. Absence of a uterus (male genotype)

499. Hypertension

500. Salt-losing crisis

Perinatology
Genetics

Answers

473. The answer is D. *(Goodwin, p 58.)* The karyotype presented consists of 47 chromosomes; in addition to a normal female genotype (46,XX) there is an extra number-16 chromosome. Although trisomy 16 has not been observed in liveborn children, it is the most common autosomal trisomy encountered in studies of spontaneous abortions. Approximately 40 percent of chromosomally abnormal abortuses are trisomic, and of these, one-quarter involve chromosome number 16.

474. The answer is E. *(Reid, p 258.)* The incidence of Turner's syndrome (45,XO) at birth is 1:3,000. In cytogenic studies of early spontaneous abortions, 45,XO chromosome constitution is detected quite frequently and accounts for approximately 20 percent of all chromosomal abnormalities detected. The vast majority (98 percent) of fetuses who have Turner's syndrome are lost prior to term; most are aborted during the first trimester.

475. The answer is D. *(Burrow, pp 835-837, 858.)* Cystic fibrosis is an autosomal recessive disorder that, until quite recently, caused death during childhood of almost all affected individuals. For the woman described in the question, the fact that two siblings were affected by cystic fibrosis indicates that her parents were both carriers for the disease. Because two-thirds of the unaffected children of couples who are both carriers for an autosomal recessive disorder also will be carriers, the woman has two chances in three of being a carrier. Assuming that her husband's family has no history of cystic fibrosis and given that the carrier frequency for this disease in the general population is 1:25, the chance that they are both carriers is (2/3 x 1/25). Because one-fourth of the children of couples who are both carriers for the same autosomal recessive disorder will have the disease, the risk that their child will be born with cystic fibrosis is (2/3 x 1/25 x 1/4), or 1:150.

476. The answer is D. *(Reid, p 258.)* A number of investigators have detected a high frequency of chromosomal abnormalities by tissue culture of first trimester abortuses. The frequency of these abnormalities is about 36 percent, of which approximately 45 percent are autosomal trisomies, 25 percent are polyploidies, and 20 percent are 45,XO. The remaining 10 percent includes autosomal monosomies, structural abnormalities, and mosaics.

477. The answer is A. *(The NICHD National Registry for Amniocentesis Study Group, JAMA 236[1976]:1471-1476.)* A national prospective controlled study, designed to evaluate the safety and accuracy of prenatal genetic diagnosis by early midtrimester amniocentesis, revealed that the incidence of fetal loss in the approximately 1,000 women studied did not differ significantly from that of the controls. As a result, the incidence of pregnancy loss directly attributable to midtrimester amniocentesis is thought to be less than 1 percent. This finding has been confirmed by a similar study conducted in Canada. The overall accuracy of midtrimester amniocentesis for prenatal genetic diagnosis was found to be 99.4 percent.

478. The answer is C. *(Goodwin, p 36.)* Only 45 chromosomes are present in the karyotype pictured. Accompanying 16 normal members of the C group (chromosome pairs 6 through 12 and the two X chromosomes) is an additional medium-size submetacentric chromosome (at the bottom center of the karyotype) similar to the C-group members. One D-group chromosome (a single member of the number-15 pair) and one G-group chromosome (a single member of the number-21 pair) are missing. The additional C-group member, thus, represents a 15,21 centric fusion chromosome. This karyotype is most consistent with a normal heterozygous carrier of a D/G translocation.

479. The answer is A (1, 2, 3). *(Speroff, p 128.)* Although monosomy of the X chromosome (45,XO) is the most common karyotype of patients who have Turner's syndrome, a variety of structural abnormalities of the X chromosome in addition to mosaics may be found in patients who have this disorder. Comparison of chromosomal abnormalities and phenotypic features in individuals who have gonadal dysgenesis indicates that the short stature and other clinical findings of the Turner's phenotype are associated with loss of the short arm of one X chromosome. Of the karyotypes listed in the question, all involve monosomy for a portion of the short arm of the X chromosome except 46,X,i(Xp). Individuals who have this karyotype have only one normal X chromosome; their other X chromosome, composed of a duplication of the normal short arm, is called an isochromosome. In essence, they are monosomic for the long arm of the X and trisomic for the short arm. This karyotype is associated with gonadal dysgenesis but not with the phenotypic features characteristic of individuals who have Turner's syndrome.

480. The answer is E (all). *(Pritchard, ed 15. pp 272-273.)* A number of methods using amniotic fluid are available for the determination during the second trimester of pregnancy of the sex of a fetus. Specific staining techniques for Barr bodies and Y chromosomes in amniotic fluid cells accurately predict fetal sex about 95 percent of the time. Testosterone levels in amniotic fluid also are very reliable indicators of fetal sex. When determination of the sex of a fetus is especially important (if, for example, the presence of an X-linked recessive disease is suspected), karyotyping of cultured amniotic fluid cells is the method of choice, because its accuracy is 99.4 percent. Sex steroid levels can confirm results obtained by the other procedures mentioned by detecting some karyotype errors due to contamination of amniotic fluid by maternal cells.

481. The answer is B (1, 3). *(Pritchard, ed 15. pp 273-274.)* The demonstration by ultrasound examination of a well-defined vertex of normal size can rule out anencephaly. Amniotic fluid levels of alpha-fetoprotein are currently the most reliable tool to detect those neural tube defects not covered by skin (open defects). Elevated levels also may be associated with fetal blood contamination of the amniotic fluid (often due to amniocentesis through an anteriorly implanted placenta) or with a number of fetal disorders. Because maternal serum alpha-fetoprotein levels have been reported to be elevated in only 50 to 70 percent of cases in which the fetus has had an open neural tube defect, its use as the exclusive diagnostic procedure in couples at increased risk for having children with this disorder is not generally recommended.

482. The answer is E (all). *(Burrow, pp 820, 859.)* X-linked dominant disorders occur more frequently in women than in men. If a man has an X-linked dominant disorder, none of his sons but all of his daughters will inherit his X chromosome; therefore all daughters will have the disease. If a woman has an X-linked dominant disorder, her children, whether female or male, will have a 50 percent chance of acquiring the affected X chromosome.

483. The answer is A (1, 2, 3). *(Speroff, p 118.)* During the early fetal life of a woman, germ cells migrate to the primitive gonad, where they rapidly proliferate by mitosis, reaching a peak of 6 to 7 million at about 20 weeks of development. Loss of germ cells begins at about 15 weeks of development, so that not more than one million remain at the time of birth. Continued loss of germ cells occurs throughout life until the menopause.

484. The answer is A (1, 2, 3). *(Thompson, ed 2. pp 149-150, 348.)* Individuals who are carriers of a balanced D/G translocation have 45 chromosomes in each cell; one D-group and one G-group chromosome have fused, forming a chromosome that resembles a member of the C group. The risk for giving birth to children who have translocation Down's syndrome is substantially higher if the wife is the carrier (10 to 12 percent) than if the husband is the carrier (2 to 3 percent). Amniocentesis can determine whether the offspring will be unaffected, will carry the translocation, or will have the disease. Because a D/G translocation can be inherited from a parent (approximately 50 percent are familial), chromosome studies of family members are recommended.

485. The answer is D (4). *(Burrow, pp 820, 859.)* If a woman who has phenylketonuria, which is an autosomal recessive disorder, marries a carrier for this disease, the chance that offspring will be affected is 50 percent. Although phenylketonuria cannot be detected prenatally, screening of newborns and early institution of low-phenylalanine diets have made it possible for affected individuals to reach adulthood. It has become apparent that a high frequency of mental retardation exists in children of mothers who have phenylketonuria, even if these children do not themselves have the disease. Retardation in these children presumably is related to intrauterine exposure to high phenylalanine levels in the maternal blood.

486-490. The answers are: 486-D, 487-E, 488-B, 489-A, 490-E. *(Burrow, pp 817, 832, 842-843, 852, 855-859, 861.)* Huntington's chorea is an autosomal dominant disorder causing progressive mental deterioration and eventual dementia. It has its clinical onset during the late reproductive years or following the reproductive years. The chance that the woman described in the question has inherited the gene from her father is 1:2. The chance that she will transmit the gene to her child also is 1:2. Therefore, the chance that her child will inherit the disease is 25 percent (1/2 x 1/2 = 1/4).

The frequency of Tay-Sachs disease is markedly higher among American Jews of Ashkenazi descent than in the general U.S. population. Screening studies indicate that the carrier frequency for the Tay-Sachs gene in this ethnic group is approximately 1:30, making the incidence of the disease 1:3,600 (1/30 x 1/30 x 1/4). Carrier testing and prenatal diagnosis can help detect the presence of the disease in a fetus and therefore provide a basis for deciding whether to continue the pregnancy.

Although the recurrence rate for trisomy 21 (Down's syndrome) is not well defined, it generally is stated to be 1 percent. This figure is based on documented recurrences in families in which one parent has a low-percentage mosaicism for a cell line with a 47,XX,+21 or 47,XY,+21 chromosome constitution. In one series of prenatal diagnoses, five trisomic fetuses were discovered in 485 pregnancies examined for Down's syndrome. The risk for having a child with Down's syndrome is not known to be increased in other relatives of children who have a primary trisomy (47,XX,+21 or 47,XY,+21). When a patient has a family history of Down's syndrome, chromosome analysis should be performed to determine if the disease is a sporadic event (primary trisomy) or a translocation. If the affected family member has translocation Down's syndrome, a chromosome study of that child's parents, relatives, or both is indicated to ascertain whether the translocation is familial or a chance event.

Neural tube defects follow a multifactorial mode of inheritance. When there have been sufficient data for the derivation of empiric risk figures, the risk for having a child with a neural tube defect has been found to increase with the birth of each affected child. The risk following the birth of one child with a neural tube defect is 3 to 5 percent; the risk following the birth of the second affected child is 12 to 13 percent. Prenatal diagnosis, based on the amniotic fluid level of alpha-fetoprotein as well as on other adjunctive studies, is available.

491-495. The answers are: 491-A, 492-A, 493-A, 494-C, 495-D. *(Pritchard, ed 15. pp 81-84.)* In the female gonad the development of primary oocytes is arrested in the first meiotic division during fetal life. This process, which is completed only at the time of mature follicular development and ovulation, results in a reduction in the number of chromosomes. Nondisjunction causes chromosomes to be distributed unequally to daughter cells during cellular division and may occur during the first or second division of meiosis as well as during mitosis. In contrast to oogenesis, there is no prolonged arrest of either meiotic division during spermatogenesis.

496-500. The answers are: 496-C, 497-B, 498-C, 499-A, 500-D. *(Speroff, pp 126-129.)* Both the androgen insensitivity syndrome and congenital adrenal hyperplasia due to a deficiency of C-17 hydroxylase result in phenotypic female development in individuals who have a 46,XY chromosome constitution. In the androgen insensitivity syndrome (testicular feminization), testosterone receptors are unable to respond normally to androgen; thus, production of estrogens by the gonads results in feminization at puberty. Because individuals who have a C-17 hydroxylase defect are unable to produce sex steroids, they do not develop secondary sexual characteristics at puberty. In both disorders, production of an inhibiting factor by the fetal testicular gonads blocks uterus formation. Deficiency in C-17 hydroxylase causes excessive production of salt-retaining corticosteroids and may lead to hypertension and hypokalemia.

Bibliography

Adamsons, K., Jr., and Joelsson, I. "The effects of pharmacologic agents upon the fetus and newborn." *American Journal of Obstetrics and Gynecology* 96 (1966):437-460.

Aladjem, S., and Brown, A.K. *Clinical Perinatology.* St. Louis: C.V. Mosby Co., 1974.

Alderman, M.H., and Schoenbaum, E.E. "Detection and treatment of hypertension at the work site." *New England Journal of Medicine* 293(1975):65-68.

American College of Obstetricians and Gynecologists. "Suspect rape." *American College of Obstetricians and Gynecologists Technical Bulletin* 14(1972): July.

American Medical Association Committee on Human Sexuality. *Human Sexuality.* Chicago: American Medical Association, 1972.

Beck. W.S. *Hematology.* Cambridge: M.I.T. Press, 1973.

Behrman, S.J., and Kistner, R.W., eds. *Progress in Infertility.* 2nd ed. Boston: Little, Brown & Co., 1975.

Benirschke, K. "Twin placenta in perinatal mortality." *New York State Journal of Medicine* 61(1961):4499-4508.

Bock, K.D. "Connection between antihypertensive drugs and disorders of potency." *German Medical Monthly* 13(1968):449-450.

Brady, L.W.; Lewis, G.C.; Antoniades, J.; et al. "Evolution of radiotherapeutic techniques." *Gynecologic Oncology* 2(1974):314-323.

Burrow, G.N., and Ferris, T.F., eds. *Medical Complications During Pregnancy.* Philadelphia: Columbia Broadcasting System, W.B. Saunders Co., 1975.

Butler, N.R.; Goldstein, H.; and Ross, E.M. "Cigarette smoking in pregnancy: Its influence on birth weight and perinatal mortality." *British Medical Journal* 2(1972):127-130.

Dickinson, R.L. *Human Sex Anatomy.* Huntington: Robert E. Krieger Publishing Co. Inc., 1949.

Dickinson, R.L., and Pierson, H.H. "The average sex life of American women." *Journal of the American Medical Association* 85(1925):1113-1117.

DiSaia, P.J.; Morrow, C.P.; and Townsend, D.E. *Synopsis of Gynecologic Oncology.* New York: John Wiley & Sons Inc., 1975.

Ellenberg, M. "Impotence in diabetics: The neurologic factor." *Annals of Internal Medicine* 75(1971): 213-219.

Golbus, M.S. "The antenatal detection of genetic disorders. Current status and future prospects." *Obstetrics and Gynecology* 48(1976): 497-506.

Goodman, L.S., and Gilman, A. *The Pharmacological Basis of Therapeutics.* 5th ed. New York: Macmillan Publishing Co. Inc., 1975.

Goodwin, J.W., et al. *Perinatal Medicine.* Baltimore: Williams & Wilkins Co., 1976.

Green, R. *Human Sexuality: A Health Practitioner's Text.* Baltimore: Williams & Wilkins Co., 1974.

Green, T.H., Jr. *Gynecology: Essentials of Clinical Practice.* 3rd ed. Boston: Little, Brown & Co., 1977.

Gunning, J.E. "The DES story." *Obstetrical and Gynecological Survey.* 31 (1976): 827-833.

Herbst, A.L.; Scully, R.E.; and Robboy, S.J. "Vaginal adenosis and other diethylstilbestrol-related abnormalities." *Clinical Obstetrics and Gynecology* 18(1975): 185-194.

Hilgers, R.D., and Lewis, J.L. "Gestational trophoblastic neoplasms." *Gynecologic Oncology* 2(1974): 460-475.

Hon, E.H. *An Atlas of Fetal Heart Rate Patterns.* New Haven: Harty Press Inc., 1968.

Ingemarsson, I. "Effect of terbutaline on premature labor. A double-blind placebo-controlled study." *American Journal of Obstetrics and Gynecology* 125(1976): 520-524.

Kistner, R.W. *Gynecology: Principles and Practice.* 2nd ed. Chicago: Year Book Medical Publishers Inc., 1971.

Kolodny, R.C. "Sexual dysfunction in diabetic females." *Diabetes* 20(1971): 557-559.

Kolodny, R.C. *Workshop in Human Sexuality at Reproductive Biology Foundation.* St. Louis: October, 1976.

Lief, H.I. *Medical Aspects of Human Sexuality: Answers to Questions by 502 Authorities.* Baltimore: Williams & Wilkins Co., 1975.

MacMahon, B. "High risk factors for endometrial cancer." *Gynecologic Oncology* 2(1974): 122-129.

Masters, W.H., and Johnson, V.E. *Human Sexual Inadequacy.* Boston: Little, Brown & Co., 1970.

Masters, W.H. and Johnson, V.E. *Human Sexual Response.* Boston: Little, Brown & Co., 1966.

McCrann, D.J., and Schifrin, B.S. "Fetal monitoring in high risk pregnancy." *Clinics in Perinatology* 1(1974):229-252.

Monif, G.R., ed. *Infectious Diseases in Obstetrics and Gynecology.* New York: Harper & Row Publishers Inc., Harper Medical Department, 1974.

Nahmias, A.J., et al. "Perinatal risk associated with maternal genetic herpes simplex virus infection." *American Journal of Obstetrics and Gynecology* 110 (1971):825.

Novak, E.R., and Woodruff, J.D. *Novak's Gynecologic and Obstetric Pathology: With Clinical and Endocrine Relations.* 7th ed. Philadelphia: Columbia Broadcasting System, W.B. Saunders Co., 1974.

Patten, B.M. *Human Embryology.* 3rd ed. New York: McGraw-Hill Book Co., Blakiston Publications, 1968.

Pillay, V.K. "Some side-effects of alpha-methyldopa." *South African Medical Journal* 50(1976):625-626.

Pritchard, J.A., and MacDonald, P.C. *Williams Obstetrics.* 15th ed. New York: Prentice-Hall Inc., Appleton-Century-Crofts Medical, 1976.

Queenan, J.T. *Modern Management of the RH Problem.* New York: Harper & Row Publishers Inc., Harper Medical Department, 1967.

Ratnoff, O.D., ed. *Treatment of Hemorrhagic Disorders.* New York: Harper & Row Publishers Inc., Harper Medical Department, 1968.

Reid, D.E., et al. *Principles and Management of Human Reproduction.* Philadelphia: Columbia Broadcasting System, W.B. Saunders Co., 1972.

Robertson, J.G. "Twin pregnancy: Morbidity and fetal mortality." *Obstetrics and Gynecology* 23(1964):330-337.

Romney, S.L., et al. *Gynecology and Obstetrics: The Health Care of Women.* New York: McGraw-Hill Book Co., Blakiston Publications, 1975.

Rutledge, F.; Boronow, R.C.; and Wharton, J.T. *Gynecologic Oncology.* New York: John Wiley & Sons Inc., 1976.

Scott, J.R. "Report on Rh immune globulin therapy." *Contemporary Obstetrics and Gynecology* 8(1976):27.

Smith, J.P., and Rutledge, F. "Advances in chemotherapy for gynecologic cancer." *Cancer* 36(1975):669-674.

Speroff, L.; Glass, R.H.; and Kase, N.G. *Clinical Gynecologic Endocrinology and Infertility.* Baltimore: Williams & Wilkins Co., 1973.

Te Linde, R.W., and Mattingly, R.F. *Operative Gynecology.* 4th ed. Philadelphia: J.B. Lippincott Co., 1970.

The NICHD National Registry for Amniocentesis Study Group. "Midtrimester amniocentesis for prenatal diagnosis." *Journal of the American Medical Association* 236(1976):1471-1476.

Thompson, J.S., and Thompson, M.V. *Genetics in Medicine.* 2nd ed. Philadelphia: Columbia Broadcasting System, W.B. Saunders Co., 1973.

Thorn, G.W., et al., eds. *Harrison's Principles of Internal Medicine.* 8th ed. New York: McGraw-Hill Book Co., Blakiston Publications, 1977.

U.S. Department of Health, Education and Welfare. *The Health Consequences of Smoking.* Washington: U.S. Department of Health, Education and Welfare, 1973.

Villee, C.A.; Villee, D.B.; and Zuckerman, A. *Respiratory Distress Syndrome: Based on a Conference at Dedham, Mass. May 1973.* New York: Academic Press Inc., 1973.

Williams, R.H., ed. *Textbook of Endocrinology.* 5th ed. Philadelphia: Columbia Broadcasting System, W.B. Saunders Co., 1974.

Williams, W.J., et al. *Hematology.* New York: McGraw-Hill Book Co., Blakiston Publications, 1972.

Wynn, R.M. *Obstetrics and Gynecology: The Clinical Core.* Philadelphia: Lea & Febiger, 1974.

Young, R.C. "Chemotherapy of ovarian cancer: Past and present." *Seminars in Oncology* 2(1975):267-276.

NOTES

NOTES